WHO WE ARE....
IS WHAT WE OFFER

Richard
Roger Statten

Just Notice ...
Just This

The Body and Mind
of the Yogas

Richard Stathem

Cover Photo: R. Stathem. Wichita Mountains Wildlife Refuge, Lawton, Oklahoma

ISBN 0-7414-3250-1

Published by:

INFINITY
PUBLISHING.COM
1094 New Dehaven Street, Suite 100
West Conshohocken, PA 19428-2713
Info@buybooksontheweb.com
www.buybooksontheweb.com
Toll-free (877) BUY BOOK
Local Phone (610) 941-9999
Fax (610) 941-9959

Printed in the United States of America
Printed on Recycled Paper
Published July 2006

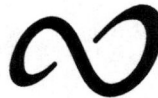

Dedication

I dedicate this book
to four personal experiences
of the early '70s that launched
my yogic journey:

I was given a copy of
Andrew Weil's
"The Natural Mind"

I discovered Billie Gollnick's
School of Yoga
in Houston, Texas

David Carradine's
television show,
Kung Fu
debuted

I was incredibly
depressed then;
thus, my heart and mind
were wide, wide open

Contents

Contents
Continued...

Part II: The Mind of Yoga

The Philosophies of Yoga

Contents
Continued...

*"Even to be attached
to the idea of enlightenment
is to go astray."*

     *Hsin Hsin
     Third Patriarch of Zen*

YOGA

Overview

1) The primary purpose of a yoga practice is to learn to *relax*. Tension is not our enemy, for muscular tension is essential to all bodily movement; however, in yoga we learn to release unnecessary tension so that we may experience life fully and *joy*fully.

2) Yoga **IS** a set of systems which enable one to comprehend and understand daily realities. Ultimately, each individual must personally decide specifically which methods to practice. In class, methods are simply *presented;* ultimately, however, each student must decide which of these methods is appropriate for personal practice.

3) Yoga is **NOT**: a religion, an escape, nor a competition.

4) Techniques taught in this book include gentle physical exercises, breathing exercises, and simple meditation methods which enable the mind to focus and concentrate.

5) ANY technique is only as effective as our willingness to practice it. Here you will learn the "how to", but if a regular, personal routine is not established, only *knowledge* will be gained ... neither wisdom nor results will be realized.

6) Be **UN**concerned with how "well" you're doing. Constantly monitoring your "progress" will only result in judgment and disappointment. If you are working to the best of your ability, then you *are* succeeding. Results come steadily and surely ... but slowly.

7) In the practice of yoga, we learn to distinguish between that which is within our conscious control and that which is "given" ... that which is just *The Way It Is*. We work with the variables and accept the constants.

8) The philosophy of yoga is that truth exists everywhere and in many traditions. No specific belief system is advanced in this book.

9) Eating should be limited to a light meal at least two hours before a Hatha Yoga (exercise) practice.

10) Before beginning work with the twists and stretches, take a minute or two to just sit or stand and focus the mind on the moment ... *in* the moment. Bring the mind to Just This ... just what is happening in the here and now ... and Just Notice. Then, with fluidity and grace-ful ... grace-filled ... movements, with full awareness on just what you're doing, begin to enter into your practice.

JUST NOTICE ... JUST THIS

The Body and Mind
of the Yogas

Introduction

This book is an introduction to the yogas ... intended to provide an understanding of the general principles of yoga for the novice, and to reinforce and further the understanding of the adept. Hopefully it will explain many of the basic terms, concepts, and ideas associated with this ancient art of body, mind, and spirit. The reader may also have noticed that the title of this book, and the title of this section of the book, refers not to yoga in the singular, but rather in the plural, because yoga is a *set* of systems consisting of many methods that, when practiced over time, enable one to learn to be *in* the moment and to discover *who* in truth we are.

The philosophy of yoga is a here-and-now philosophy. Put simply, yoga enables one to discover that the body is what we have, not who we are. Perhaps the most common misconception of yoga is that it is mainly an exercise system. It's true that the yogas include a very sophisticated exercise system ... called Hatha Yoga ... but yoga, in its true, broad sense, is much more than that. Yoga teaches us how to be with what is, and how to work constructively with whatever the moment has to offer ... regardless of our personal feelings about it and irrespective of dogma.

The language of yoga is Sanskrit. The terminology and descriptive phrases common to the discipline of yoga originated in this ancient, eastern language. The far-eastern Sanskrit, like the western Latin, is no longer in common use; however, it is the language that labels and identifies the techniques of yoga. In order to familiarize the reader with the language of yoga, Sanskrit terms, along with their English translations, are used in this book.

The word "YOGA" is a Sanskrit word which literally means "union". What is "united" in yoga varies with the level and the type of practice. "Yoga" may refer to the union of interpersonal relationships, union between the various physiological systems of the body, union between the many psychological systems of the mind, union and integration between mind and body, or the union between one's worldly self and the vast, nameless Spiritual Essence. "Yoga" refers to the joining together, the uniting, of all of the many "selves" and identities we all have ... like the hub connects the spokes of a wheel ... and as the wheel's rim surrounds it all. In our daily yoga practice, which includes *all* that the day offers, we focus on the **philosophy** of yoga. Yoga philosophy is neither "eastern" nor "western" ... it is universal ... as stated in the title of this book: "just notice ... just this". Above all else, yoga is a philosophy of *common sense* ... a philosophy of *being in the moment.* Yoga philosophy holds that we are whole and complete just as we are, but many of us have lost touch with an awareness of that perfection by becoming attached to the ***things*** of this world ... including (and especially) attachment to, and identification with, the body. Yoga awareness reveals that suffering originates with *attachments.* There is nothing we must *get*, for we *are* it all already ... but we must learn to create an environment in which we can realize what it is we already have ... and what and who we truly *are*.

This process of *re*-membering ... re-joining ... re-yoking ... can be likened to the slow, steady process of peeling back veils covering a bright light. The veils do not determine whether or not the light shines, nor even how brightly it shines. The veils do, however, prevent us from *seeing* the light ... and prevent the light from *revealing.* The "veils" of our mind include our psychological attachments, which manifest as ignorance, confusion, fear, laziness, and anger ... and which prevent us from experiencing the Light(ness) of our true being. And the Light(ness) of our true state of being is Happiness ... Pure Joy! It is ours for the taking!

The eastern word "yoga", like the western word "education", implies a very broad and general reference. "Yoga" refers not to *one* method or practice, but rather to a ***set of systems*** which, when fully applied, result in complete and total awareness of True Self. As we become aware of True Self, we no longer have to *believe* we are/have a Soul ... as we experience that truth, it becomes *known.* What is known needn't be believed, just as we don't have to "believe" in gravity because we experience the truth of it every moment of every day.

The yoga of physical exercise and body work is called *Hatha* Yoga. This is the yoga most Westerners perceive as "yoga" ... period. Many believe Hatha Yoga to be the sum total of yoga. Yoga indeed does include physical stretching and twisting exercises, as well as breathing exercises; however, to consider Hatha Yoga as *all* of yoga is like considering physical education in school to be *all* of education. The work with the body is only the *beginning* of the work of yoga. Having said that, it's true that this book devotes many pages to Hatha Yoga ... the beginning work of yoga ... the physical exercises of yoga. Nevertheless, the techniques presented here will enable the practitioner to link the body work with the mind work. They *are*, in truth, inseparable. All of the practices of yoga include a "mind set" that is all too often absent from today's wide assortment of exclusively physical-health-related methods.

Although a yoga practice usually includes Hatha Yoga, for the purpose of creating and maintaining a comfortable and functional body, the work also includes the breathing techniques of Pranayam Yoga ... to provide the body with the essential elixir of life (oxygen ... referred to in yoga as "prana") and to rhythmically couple the systems of mind and body. The work also includes the Raja Yoga of simple, concentrative, meditation methods to harmonize the energies of Being, and to quiet and focus the mind ... that it may become a powerful and effective instrument. Additionally, the work encompasses the development of the intellect through Jnana Yoga, and a heightened sense of purpose and meaning to life through service in Karma Yoga. We may also choose to discover and explore the essence of our Spiritual Nature with the practice of Bhakti and/or Satsang (churchly worship) Yoga. Several major systems, in addition to Hatha Yoga, comprise the techniques enabling one to lift the veils of *maya* ... the veils of illusion. (Indeed, the mind and philosophy systems of yoga existed for more than 600 years before the exercise systems of Hatha Yoga were created). Some of these systems are briefly described and defined in the following section of this book.

In the practice of the yogas we assume and accept full responsibility for our current state of being, even as we begin the gentle, systematic process of flowing through our practice in positive directions. Harmony is our natural state! These methods help us learn to create an environment in which this natural, harmonious condition may be realized.

When practicing the methods of yoga we learn to gently release clinging to how we **want** the world to be ... and begin to see it ... and even *accept* it! ... **as it is**. We learn to work with what **is**, and we begin to understand **why** it is as it is.

Relaxation is the essence of a yoga practice. The practitioner learns to relax at two levels: the work with body and mind techniques enables 1) the release of physical tensions and emotional stresses that manifest in the body in the course of a day. But, more profoundly, the practitioner also learns 2) to perceive the world from an *enlightened* perspective of consciousness and awareness so that the usual daily stresses and tensions are much less likely to manifest at all. Tension is not our enemy, for muscle tension is necessary to body movement; however, in yoga we learn to release unnecessary tension so that we may experience life fully and *joy*fully.

So far, I have been telling you what yoga IS! ... a set of systems enabling us to comprehend, understand, and work with the realities of the day. In this book, methods are simply *presented;* however, each of us must decide which of these methods is appropriate for our own personal practice. So many misconceptions surround yoga that it is helpful to also examine what yoga is *not* ...

Yoga is **NOT** a religion! Religions advise acceptable behavior and suggest what is *"beyond"* worldly existence ... and how to get there. Yoga is a philosophy which advises us how to **be** ... in *this* world and in *this* time. As friend and colleague, Tulsa acupuncturist and Jin Shin Juitzu Master, Mark Hovis, once said, "We are human BE-ings Not human BECOM-ings!" We are whole and complete just as we are. We are at once *perfect* as we are, and yet with much shaping and forming and work to do. Yoga teaches us to work with what *is* … and *how* to work with what is.

Yoga is **NOT** an escape! It's tempting and easy, once a practice is established, to want to escape into that practice … to use it to avoid duties and responsibilities … to *prefer* it to the stuff of the day. But the purpose of a practice in the first place is to learn to work *with* the stuff of life. In time, and as our practice deepens, we discover that, not only is there no escaping the responsibilities of daily life, there is not even a *need* to escape from anything, nor even anything to escape from! Events of the day become challenges and opportunities rather than threats or affronts.

Yoga is **NOT** a competition! In our yoga practice we are simply creating an environment in which results reveal themselves. Focusing on results is one of the first, and often the most terminal, of the "games" the mind plays on the practicing self, because the results are never soon enough, nor quantitative enough, nor often are they even what we thought they should be in the first place. Therefore, we compete with no one … not even with our self. *Especially* not with our self! All we're doing in our practice is creating an environment … just creating an environment in which our BE-ing can unfold. Like planting a seed: we can't actually *grow* a plant. We can't reach into the seed and pull out and shape the stems and the leaves and the roots and *make* it grow! Not even if we want to … it can't be done … it's not an option. But what we can do is create an environment in which the plant *can* grow strong and healthy … a nourishingly controlled environment, not a restrictively controlled one. So it is with our practice. All we're doing is creating the environment. It's all we *can* do … it's all we *need* do.

Until now, the word "practice" has been used primarily as a noun … as in referencing "Our Practice". But "practice" is also a verb … practice is what we *do*, as well as what we create. *We practice our practice!* Vivekananda spoke a pure and simple truth when he said, "You may sit and read or listen to lectures by the hour, but if there is no *practice*, there will be no progress. You will go no further." Studying the methods is good and useful, but *practice* is absolutely essential. In the early stages, we set aside time to practice, but what eventually evolves is amazing: we discover that **our whole life is our practice!** That every event of every day is "sadhana" … method … technique … that takes us closer and closer to our goal of Self discovery.

In the practice of yoga, we learn to distinguish between that which is within our conscious control and that which is "given" … that which is just *The Way It Is*. We learn to work with the variables and accept the constants. It's that simple. It's not always that *easy* … but it's just that simple!

The Varieties of Yoga

As mentioned in the ***Introduction***, Hatha Yoga is the exercise system of yoga, and it is an essential focus of this book. However, in practicing the stretching and twisting exercises of Hatha Yoga, other yogas should complement the Hatha practice as well. Indeed, the execution of the physical exercises of Hatha Yoga alone is not truly practicing "yoga" ... the other yogas must be a part of the practice.

The following is a brief list and description of some of the yogas that, although perhaps less familiar than the exercises of Hatha, are just as essential to a yoga practice. Some will be discussed in greater depth later in this book.

1) **JNANA** (pronounced "ja-na" or "n'ya-na") – is the yoga of intellect ... development of the mind. Jnana Yoga includes studies and academic pursuits, and general mind development in the acquisition of knowledge.

2) **VIPASANA** – is the meditation practice of *passive observation*. This essential yoga employs simply noticing one's outer and inner environments passively ... without judgment or definition. It is a perfect complement to Hatha Yoga! As one *just notices* the sense-sations of the moment (such as the body's posture), the mind is gently brought into the present ... the "now". It is said in yoga that the one true time is *now* and the one true place is *here*. Vipasana, an amazingly simple, yet quite challenging, practice teaches us to rest in and discover the truth of the moment.

3) **DHARMA** – referred to as the "right path", is discovering one's natural, innate skills and talents ... and *practicing* them, utilizing them, and offering them to others ... simply through the practice. It is said that the only thing we can truly offer another being is *our* being. As we discover our dharma, we discover our talents and exploit them in a positive way to help en-lighten the world. One's dharma may manifest as being a business person, or a teacher, or a homemaker, and expressing those talents in the form of *service*. The crucial issue is *how* the dharma is practiced, not the form the dharma takes. Appearances can be deceiving! The practice of the yogas may include any activity that is positive, constructive, and enlightening.

4) **KARMA** – has many meanings in yoga, including "right action". In this context, karma relates to *how* one's dharma is practiced. Karma means performing the tasks that make up one's dharma without focusing on the goals or rewards of the actions, but rather, acting purely and simply for the sake and pleasure of the acts themselves. (Karma does not mean that one does not accept payment or reward for actions, but simply that those are not the goals and focus of the actions.)

5) **RAJA** – means "kingly" and generally refers to the many meditation methods that enable control and focus of mind energy. Vipasana, mentioned above, is a practice of

Raja Yoga ... as is mantra (sound) meditation and yantra (visual) meditation and the many meditation practices that incorporate the breathing techniques ("prana" yoga ... see below).

6) **BHAKTI** - the yoga of spiritual devotion. This yoga may include the gathering together of like-minded individuals to practice churchly worship (satsang), or it may be practiced in solitude. Bhakti Yoga enables the practitioner to discover and honor the spiritual nature of all things ... *including* the things that one may not personally like!

8) **PRANA** – generally refers to the breathing practices of yoga, but the word "prana" actually means "life force". It also encompasses the nutrition we ingest in the form of food for the body. But since breathing is on-going, prana is sometimes considered synonymous with breath. Various breathing exercises (several of which are discussed later in this book) enable the student of yoga to learn to control and direct the energies of mind and body.

All of the practices of the yogas overlap and encompass one another ... none exist in a vacuum ... and each is based in *practicality* and purpose. This sometimes surprises the beginning student, who may initially think of yoga as other-worldly or esoteric. As previously mentioned, yoga is **not** an escape. Yoga teaches one how to be in the world as effectively and constructively as is humanly possible ... to discover, through the mundane truth of being human, that this life *is* the "spiritual experience"! That *this* is the experience of spirituality manifest in material form. And as our attachments to the ever-transient material forms lighten, our appreciation for the material forms deepens. The paradoxes one discovers in the practice are not only fascinating, amazing, and sometimes surprising, they are also often even a source of humor! Humor is an important part of the work of yoga.

Before we can effectively work to deepen consciousness and awareness, we must first know where we currently *are* ... psychologically as well as physically ... then proceed systematically, gently, and consciously. The techniques of yoga are specifically structured to help facilitate this conscious unfolding. In time, and **with practice**, we discover that there is, indeed, nothing to "accomplish" ... we are already the essence of accomplishment. We are simply DIScovering (UNcovering) who, *in truth*, we already are! We practice the methods as a means of peeling back the thin, numerous veils of ignorance that separate us from truth ... from pure joy ... from the immortality of Spirit. We begin to perceive all of the events of life as continuous, enlightening Acts of Grace ... as sadhana ... as opportunities to deepen the work ... to enhance the en(ner)-light-enment ... to personally discover and realize the truth of Thomas Aquinas' words:

*"Service
is the highest
form of prayer."*

VIPASANA – MEDITATION

(Just Noticing)

The Vipasana technique of meditation, mentioned in *The Varieties of Yoga*, deserves some elaboration because it creates a mindset essential to the practice of Hatha and other yogas. It also creates a mindset essential to moving through the experiences of the day. Vipasana is a here-and-now practice that embodies the very meaning of *yoga*.

Meditation is the process of becoming aware. It begins as a verb ... as a practice ... as something *done*; in time it becomes a noun ... a state of being ... a *way* of being. In its various stages of practice, meditation affects consciousness at many levels.

For instance, at the "level" ("levels" should not be perceived on a hierarchy as "high" or "low", but rather simply as differing mental states that equally *co*-exist. All "levels" of being are considered valid and relevant) of ordinary waking consciousness, meditation is an exercise that teaches the mind to focus and concentrate. A regular, disciplined meditation practice creates a powerful and functional mind. As we learn to focus mental energy, all tasks ... in the workplace, driving a car, interpersonal relationships ... are performed more effectively and efficiently. At this level, a regular and consistent meditation practice is also very *practical*.

At another level, meditation enables a state of rest so deep and complete that even while consciously in the body and the world, we begin to *experience* the distinction between the body, which inhabits the world, and the **Self**, which inhabits the body. We discover that the body is not who we *are* ... it is what we *have*.

Meditation enables one to bridge the gap between the *believed* ... and the *known*.

The technique presented here is generally referred to as Contemplative Meditation, Zen Meditation, or Vipasana Meditation. With this technique, one practices *passively* observing ("just noticing") the immediate environment. It is this *just noticing* that, in time and with practice, enables the deep relaxation that creates an environment in which the truth that is already ours can simply rise to the surface of our consciousness and be known.

As the student sits in comfortable balance, the body's *sense*-sations are passively observed ... just noticed: the tactile sensations, the movement of breath in the nostrils and throughout the body, the variety of sounds, the light falling on the eyelids, the rising and passing thoughts. There is no attempt to classify, categorize, or evaluate these sense-sations; they are merely observed ... *simply* observed ... **Just Noticed.**

This *just noticing* is a very simple, yet powerful, method. It enables one to begin releasing the attachments that accompany the judging, anticipating, and evaluating mind so we can open to the teaching and learning experiences inherent in each moment ... rather than continually coloring every experience with our wants-and-desires. It is a method so simple that its very simplicity tends to confound a mind that has come to believe that the process of living *must be* complicated and complex, rather than natural, easy, and flowing.

We must slowly grow into this new way of being. Thus, a regular, consistent practice is essential. In time the mind becomes calm and centered ... an *instrument* of the Self rather than its dictator. The Hatha Yoga practice, too, takes on a profound meaning much deeper than mere physical exercise.

The Method -

1) If possible, set a timer. (Five to ten minutes is a good start.)

2) Sit comfortably ... either on the floor, or sit in a straight-backed chair with legs un-crossed and the feet flat on the floor.

3) Envelop the body with conscious awareness by taking a moment to quietly observe the senses and *just notice* the stimuli ... without judgment ... as if inhabiting a body for the first time ... as if the experience were new and unique. **Feel** the clothing against the skin, *just notice* the smells, the sounds, the light falling on the eyelids, tastes, etc.

4) After passively observing the senses for several moments, let the awareness come to rest on one physical sensation, such as the gentle abdominal rise and fall in harmony with the breath, or the physical sensation of the air flowing into and out of the nostrils. Let that sensation serve as a *point of focus* for the mind. (Note: The specific sensation selected is not important, but it **is** important to work with **that** focal point continually ... for at least several months. Changing the focal point frequently just agitates the mind and tends to result in an obsession with "getting results", rather than just working, regularly, without judgment and without expectations.)

5) Simply observe ... *just notice* ... the chosen focal point for the duration of the practice. If the mind wanders (and it will!), simply return it to its focal point ... time and time again ... as often as necessary ... **without judgment**. It is the nature of the mind to wander (after all, it's had fairly free rein to do so most of its life!), but now we are training it to focus and concentrate, and we must direct it with the same consistent compassion and firm resolve with which we would direct a child's actions.

6) When the timer sounds, *terminate the meditation.* If the sitting has been particularly relaxing and pleasant, it may be tempting to extend the practice time; or if the mind is particularly agitated at the outset, we may be tempted to forego practice altogether. However, we must remember that the objective is not pleasure or avoidance, nor is it bliss or even relaxation ... our objective is to create a disciplined, controlled mind. And it is **un**disciplined to manipulate the practice in deference to whims and wishes.

Practice just for the sake of practice. Forget about objectives, goals, and purposes. Do not be preoccupied with results. *Just practice* ... and by so doing you will create an environment in which results *will* simply *reveal* themselves!

Creating A Practice

"You can sit, listen to lectures, and read books by the hour,
*but unless there is **practice**, you will not progress.*
Practice is absolutely necessary!"

Vivekananda

The Spirit is not the focus of the work of yoga. The body is not the focus of the work of yoga. It is the **mind** that is the focus of the work of yoga.

The Spirit, of course, *needs* no work. It certainly doesn't need *us* to improve upon it. It's perfect just as it is. And as preoccupied as most westerners are with body image (and it's becoming even more so!), it's no small wonder that if most people are asked if they "do yoga", they will think and reply in terms of physical exercise. But it's the mind that becomes confused ... early in life (in large part because of what and how it's taught) ... and it's the tangled mind that we seek to unravel through the practice we create. We accomplish this, ironically enough, in large part through work with the body! Thus, the body is not only the physical vehicle of the Self, it also becomes the *vehicle* of our practice ... rather like using a thorn to extract a thorn. Although we work with the body, we use the sensations (the "*sense – sations*") the body creates as a focal point for the mind. Not only does the body become a healthy and useful vehicle for the Self, it also ceases to be a distraction, as we increasingly turn the focus of our practice to reigning in, controlling, and calming the mind.

Relaxation, at two levels, is both the outer and the inner goal of our work. At one level, relaxation simply *feels* good. It certainly feels better than tension! Relaxation is pleasure, and it is pleasurable; and we discover in our practice that pleasure, free from attachment (no small feat!) is perfectly safe. At another level, we discover that as we increasingly rest in the place of relaxation (regardless of our immediate setting and circumstances), we begin to "see" the truth of the moment more clearly. We discover that those things that once created and sustained our tension, no longer throws us off center ... or, at least, not as far off center as they once did.

Having now repeatedly emphasized that the importance of the work is not the body ... let us begin the work **with the body**! This is no contradiction ... although, perhaps, somewhat of a paradox. The body is the grossest (as in "most obvious" ... not "disgusting") manifestation of the Self ... it is a manifestation ... a part ... of who we are. Therefore, it is a logical place to begin the work. It is very important to remember this: if you are practicing to the best of your ability, then you are accomplishing your objective! Yoga is absolutely, totally, and completely **non**-competitive! Not even with our self are we competing! When we stretch the muscles as effectively as we can … vigorously, *not* strenuously … we cleanse and tone the muscles. More is not better. As we stretch and twist the body, we are gently – *gently* – realigning the skeletal structure of the body. It has taken us a lifetime to get where we presently are … both mentally and physically … and the redirection must be slow and gradual … with *no* emphasis on progress! If we keep evaluating and judging our work, the results will never be quantitatively nor qualitatively enough. Instead, we simply – *simply* – create an environment in which the results can reveal themselves.

When we work with the mind to redirect the mind, it goes to work almost *instantly* to talk us out of our practice … to convince us that "life was not really so bad before, and besides, the exercises make me sore … I felt better before doing this! … and there are a lot more constructive things I could be doing right now than *this*!" We must be prepared for this … and learn to *ignore* it! The mind is very very subtle and persuasive and tricky. But eventually, the mind must learn that it can *not* want to do, but still do; and it can *want* to do, and *not* do. For instance, we can *not* want to mow the lawn, and still mow it; we can *not* want to go to work, and still go. Likewise, we can *want* a candy bar or a smoke or a drink … and not get it! We don't have to get rid of the desires; all we have to do is develop the strength to be fully aware of the desires … equally - the desires to do, and the desires to not do … then act responsibly. We no longer have to be enslaved by our wants and desires systems. It's just that simple! Of course, what is simple is not always easy, but just as we can exercise the body and develop physical strength; so, too, we can exercise the mind, and develop its strengths, powers, and will … more than we ever thought possible! The work is simple, powerful, and effective. All we have to do, like it says in the TV ad, is: just **do** it! Sound advice indeed! Now we begin the *doing* …

The physical exercises of Hatha Yoga are categorized in this book in the following routines: 1) sitting, 2) standing, 3) stomach reclining, 4) back reclining, and 5) breathing. None of these practices exist in a vacuum; they are interdependent. Nevertheless, they are first isolated into individual lessons, for the purpose of presentation, and then linked as routines … creating a continuous flow … from this … to this … to this …

Part I

The Body of Yoga

Basic Sitting Postures

The Sanskrit word for "posture" is *asana*. Hatha yoga exercises are somewhat unique from many other forms of exercise. With hath yoga, a posture is assumed for a specific physiological purpose, and maintained for the time necessary for the body to do the work on itself (usually one to three minutes). A good starting point for a practice is to simply *sit* for a moment before beginning ... taking a few minutes to bring the awareness into the moment ... into the present ... becoming conscious of the sensations and feelings of the moment ... aware of the flow of breath into and out of the body.

Proper posture is important. Posture physically creates and maintains a body's comfort level, and psychologically creates a setting for reflecting on self-perception.

Proper posture does not require that the body be stiff or rigid. However, when sitting or standing, the head, neck, and spine should be in alignment. Carrying the body with alignment assures proper functioning of internal physical systems, and psychologically it creates and conveys self esteem and confidence. Proper posture enhances body balancing and mind centering.

Body and mind learn from, and teach, one another. In yoga we practice external exercises in order to cultivate inherent inner powers. As the power of inner awareness is cultivated, we discover truth ... and our "burden" is lightened. As our burden is lightened, we begin to simultaneously feel calm and peaceful, *and* strong and powerful. As posture improves, inner awareness is cultivated ... *naturally*. With regular and continuous yoga practice, the systems of mind and body are harmonized.

SITTING

Two sitting postures are most often practiced in Hatha Yoga: the traditional cross-legged sitting posture, which includes several variations, and sitting with the legs folded under the body. Both postures work uniquely with the body, especially with the knees, and in different ways ... and both postures should be practiced regularly. However, due to such practical considerations as body structure and condition of the knees, it may be necessary to work with one of the sitting postures most often ... while not ignoring the other.

1) Cross-legged: It is sufficient to simply sit with the legs folded one before the other. Full Lotus sitting is not necessary, nor is it necessarily recommended for the beginning student ... it may be too vigorous for knees unaccustomed to such sitting. If one is beginning a yoga practice at a fairly young age, then it may be relatively easy to work into full Lotus. Otherwise, the simple "tailor" pose, as pictured here, or the half-Lotus ... with one foot on the opposite thigh ... is sufficient. What *is* important, regardless of the sitting posture selected is that the spine remain straight (slightly arched back) and the head up and in alignment with the spine.

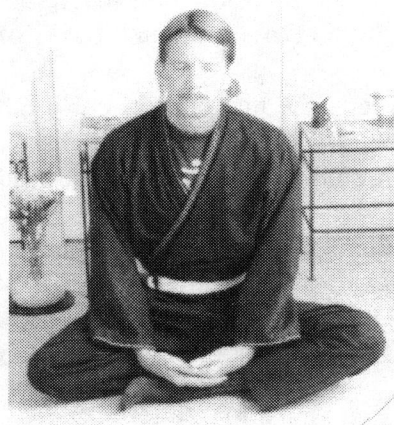

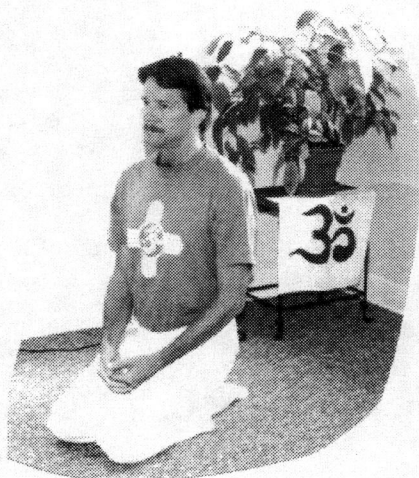

2) Vajrasana (The Diamond Pose) – is a sitting posture in which the legs are folded under, and sitting is supported by the heels. It may help to put a cushion between the legs, or under the feet, or both, to compensate for stiff knees and muscles.

It is irrelevant which sitting posture is selected, but it is important to work with *both* postures, because both sitting postures increase flexibility in the knees and ankles ... but differently. Avoid just working with the postures of your preference! Enjoy the postures you like ... but not at the expense of the others. Remember: doing the work of Life is not just doing what we like, but doing our duty ... taking responsibility. It's okay to like what we're doing, but it's not necessary.

PASHIMATANA

The Head-to-knee Pose

Pashimatana is a powerful abdominal exercise which vigorously stretches the posterior muscles ... from the achilles tendons to the back of the neck. This posture is excellent for relieving many of the tensions that manifest in the body in the course of the day, and, as such, is the ideal asana with which to follow the opening, quieting, sitting posture.

1) Sit on the floor with the spine straight and the legs extended directly in front ... knees and feet touching, and backs of the knees pressed gently, flat against the floor.

2) Place the hands atop the thighs. Exhale, then inhale deeply and completely. Let the head drop back, teeth gently touching (not clenched) so that the throat is vigorously stretched. Hold several seconds; feel the stimulation in the throat. As you exhale ...

3) Bend slowly forward from the waist. Extend the arms and hands down the sides of the legs to, or toward, the feet ... stretching forward as completely as is comfortably possible. Grasp the calves or feet, and gently pull the torso forward until you feel a vigorous, but not uncomfortable, stretch in the back and in the hamstring muscles.

Note: Be UNconcerned with the degree of stretch! If you are stretching to the best of your ability, then you are accomplishing your objective.

While breathing gently and abdominally, hold the posture for 30 seconds to a minute, initially; two to three minutes, eventually.

4) Exhale, slightly increasing the stretch, and inhale slowly as you s-l-o-w-l-y pull the body upright. *Feel* the spine as the vertebrae align ... one atop the other.

5) Place your hands behind you, palms down, fingers pointing away from the body; drop the head back, arch the spine vigorously, stretch and exhale.

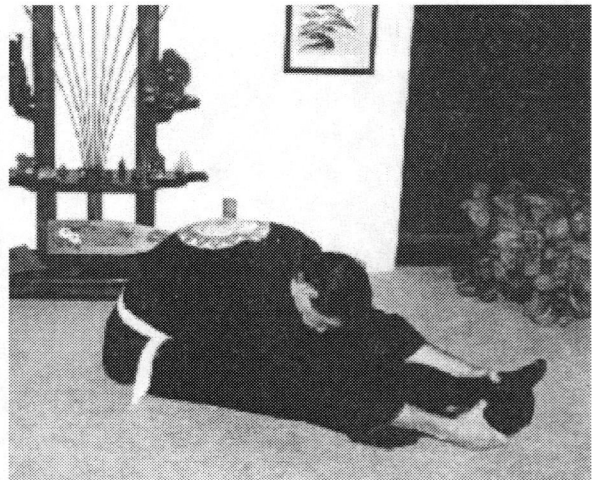

"Those who would conquer must yield;
those who conquer do so because *they yield."*

Lao Tsu

BHODI – KONASANA

The Butterfly Pose ... The Inner-thigh Stretch

Bhodi-konasana increases flexibility in the ankles and knees, and stretches and strengthens the muscles of the lower back ... in addition to vigorously stretching the muscles of the inner thighs. The Inner-thigh Stretch often follows one of the head-to-knee poses, such as Pashimatana or Janu-sirasana (next page).

1) Sit on the floor with the knees bent and the soles of the feet pressed together. Wrap the hands around the feet and draw the heels in close to the body. Inhale deeply and completely, and as you exhale, slowly ...

2) Bend forward from the waist, place the elbows in the folds of the legs, and as you pull up on the feet press firmly down on the legs ... bringing the knees as close as possible to the floor.

3) Relax the breathing and hold the posture for thirty seconds to a minute, initially ... one to three minutes, eventually.

4) Exhale, increasing the stretch slightly. On an inhalation, release the stretch and c-u-r-l the body up *slowly* from the base of the spine.

5) As you exhale, place your hands on the floor behind you, slowly straighten the legs, and arch the spine vigorously.

As you move from posture to posture, let the change and the movement also become part of the practice. *Feel* each movement ... out of an asana ... into an asana ... and become aware even of the mind directing the movements.

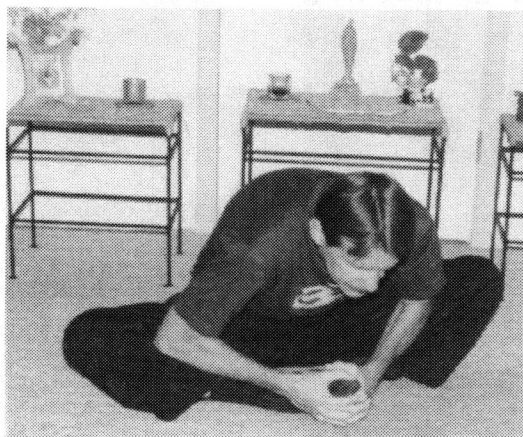

J A N U – S I R A S A N A

A head-to-knee variation

Janu-sirasana is a posture that combines the hamstring stretch of Pashimatana (head-to-knee) with the inner-thigh stretch of Bhodi-konasana (the Butterfly); however, this posture also vigorously stretches the lateral body muscles.

1) Sit with the legs extended before the body ... the same as with the starting posture for Pashimatana.

2) Bend one knee and place that foot to the inside of the thigh of the opposite leg. (If knee and ankle flexibility permit, the foot may be placed *atop* the opposite thigh.) Rest the hands slightly on each side of the extended leg.

3) Exhale completely; then inhale deeply and completely. Let the head fall back, teeth gently touching, throat stretched vigorously. Hold for a few seconds, visualizing the stimulated circulation in the throat.

4) On a slow exhalation, bend forward from the waist, extending the hands as close as possible to the outstretched foot.

5) Hold the posture 30 seconds to a minute, initially; two to three minutes eventually. As the posture is held, the breath should be gentle and abdominal ... the mind's attention should be focused on the body resting in the asana and on the physical sensations.

6) Exhale. Gradually inhale and curl the body upright. Place your hands behind you, fingers pointing away from the body, exhale and arch the spine vigorously. Release.

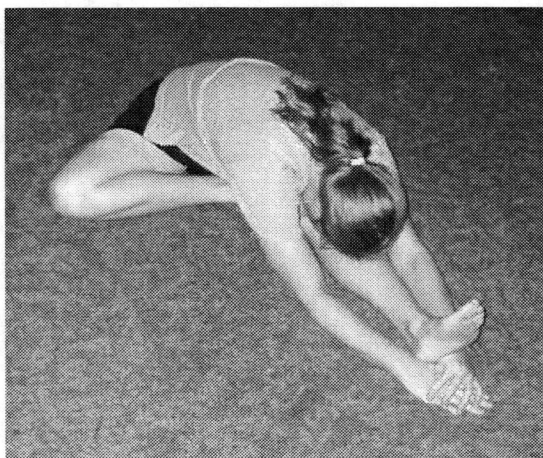

7) Repeat the procedure with the positioning of the legs reversed.

"Suffering results from our inability to distinguish between the way things are, and the way we want them to be."
                                                                    Vivekananda

YOGA NECK EXERCISES

Tension often manifests and settles in the neck and shoulders. The following simple exercise helps to relieve and release that tension. It can be practiced virtually anywhere, with no special devices, in just a few minutes. It is simple ... yet effective.

It should be mentioned, though, that muscular tension is necessary and *important,* if the body is to move and function properly. Tension is neither bad nor undesirable; however, one should be able to *release* tension once it is no longer necessary. But tension sometimes lingers, and it is this inability to *release* the tension that causes most people difficulties ... not the tension itself.

The technique:

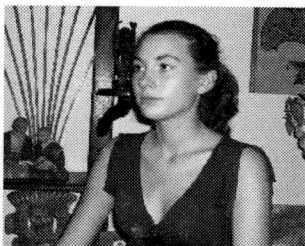

1) Sit, on the floor or in a straight-backed chair, with the head, neck, and spine in comfortable alignment. Face forward. On an exhalation, consciously relax the muscles in the face and shoulders. Inhale deeply into the abdomen. As you exhale ...

2) Let the head drop forward, bringing the chin as close as is comfortably possible to the chest. Do not let the shoulders slump. Focus the awareness on the stretching muscles in the back of the neck. Hold for about 30 seconds ... stretching vigorously, but without discomfort. On a slow inhalation, lift the head up and, as you exhale, in a continuous motion ...

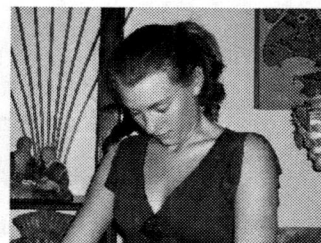

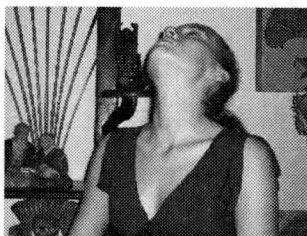

3) Let the head drop back. Vigorously stretch the throat, teeth gently touching (but not clenched). Hold the stretch about 30 seconds while focusing the awareness on the stimulated circulation in the throat: the glands, the muscles, the skin, the esophagus. On a gentle inhalation, lift the head up, and on an exhalation ...

4) Let the head drop to the left. Hold about 30 seconds, focusing awareness in the muscles on the right side of the neck. On a gentle inhalation, lift the head up, and on an exhalation ...

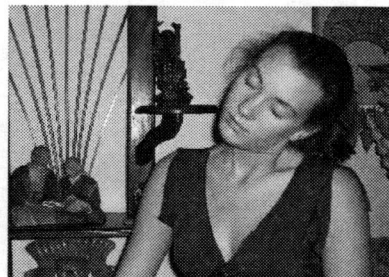

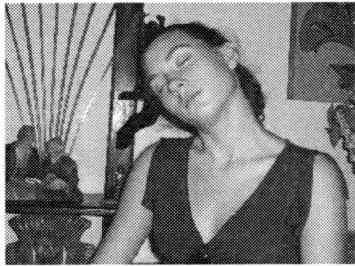

5) Let the head drop to the right. Hold 30 seconds, focusing awareness in the muscles on the left side of the neck. Gently inhale and lift the head up; on an exhalation ...

6) Drop the head forward again - chin to chest. Inhale, slowly *rotating* the head to the right, and back; exhale, rotating the head to the left, and forward again. Continue, completing three to five slow, conscious rotations. After the final rotation repeat the procedure, rotating the head in the opposite direction.

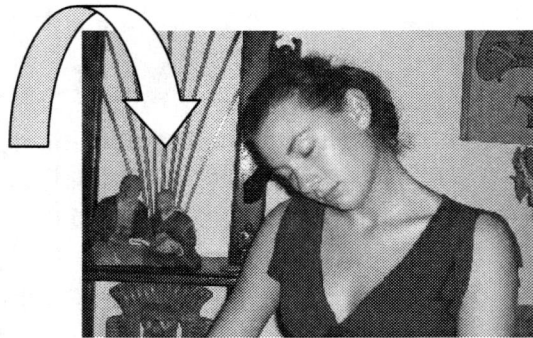

Note: 1) Initially, you may feel and hear a slight popping in the neck. This is generally due to calcium accumulation and is no cause for concern; it will diminish in time and with practice. 2) It is the *visualization* and *focusing* of the mind on the exercises that, in part, makes a yoga practice unique. In yoga we do not exercise and posture while the mind wanders elsewhere. The mind is focused in the moment ... and on the moment.

As you practice the exercises of Hatha Yoga, visualize as if the body rest at the center of a sphere, with the vision on the surface of the sphere. As the vision rotates around the body, you see it from all angles ... all sides. This simple technique will help to keep the mind *in* the moment and *on* the practice.

A R D H A – M A T S Y E N D R A S A N A

The Half Twist

Ardha-matsyendrasana creates and maintains flexibility and strength in the spine channel (Sushumna) of the body. In addition to specifically affecting the spinal system, the Half Twist also has a powerful impact on the body's nervous system ... as well as on the liver, pancreas, spleen, intestines, and kidneys. Let's begin working with the left side ...

1) Sit on the floor in a cross-legged position. Place your left hand flat on the floor behind you, close to the rear, fingers pointing away from the body.

2) Raise and position the left leg so that the left foot is flat on the floor and the left knee is upright.

3) With the right leg still flat on the floor, move it to the left and back several inches, and move the left leg so that the left foot is now on the right side of the right knee.

4) Straighten the right arm before you, and swivel it to the left side of the left knee. Lower the right arm against the left knee ... bringing the right hand down towards the left ankle, as close as possible, using the right arm as leverage against the knee.

5) Face forward. Inhale deeply and completely, and on an exhalation twist the head and body to the left as completely as possible (without straining).

6) Relax the breathing and hold the posture for 30 seconds to a minute, initially ... two to three minutes eventually.

Variation: At about the mid-time point, as you inhale, slowly swivel the head back in the opposite direction as far as possible; hold for a moment. Then, on an exhalation, swivel the head back to the posture position ... increasing the twist slightly.

7) Release the posture on an exhalation ... swiveling back to forward-facing. Reverse the positioning of the legs and arms, and repeat the posture on the other side.

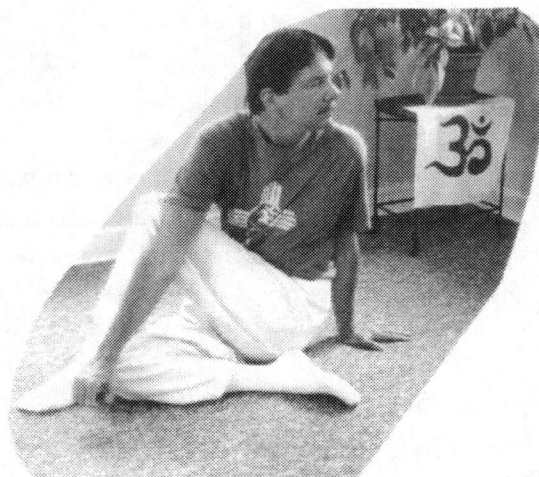

9

PRANAYAMAS

Breathing Techniques

As previously mentioned, proper breathing is important when working with the asanas ... indeed, as it is when working with every moment of every day! When practicing the postures, the movements are accompanied by appropriate and conscientious inhalations and exhalations, as described in the lessons. And when the body is at rest, the breathing should *always* be gentle and abdominal, with scarcely any upper chest movement at all.

The breathing exercises of yoga are called "pranayams" or "pranayamas" and they are considered the conscious link between the physical body, the mind, and the subtler manifestations of Self (subtle to the senses) such as soul or spiritual essence. The word "prana" refers to the sustaining life-force in the body, and it is found in food and water, as well as in breath. But the flow of breath is a continuous and conscious flow; so breathing exercises have been created to sustain and work with that flow.

Breathing is unique among systems of the body because it is the only autonomic ("involuntary") system over which we can easily assume a fairly high degree of voluntary, conscious control. In other words, most of us can hold our breath in, or out, for at least a few seconds more easily than, say, we can consciously direct our digestive system or heart rate.

The breath *mirrors* one's mental state. For instance, when listening very intently, breathing becomes still and quiet. When one is angry, the breath tends to come in short, shallow gasps. Sometimes when one is anxious or tense, the breath is retained. Yet, controlled breathing can also *establish* a mental state, as well as reflect it. Continuous slow, steady, deep breathing calms the body and mind, regardless of surrounding melodramas. However, as with all goals and achievements, *practice* is essential.

Inhalation - **puraka** - consists of two stages: first, the diaphragm expands, enabling air to fill the lower lungs; second, the diaphragm is relaxed and the chest expands, filling the upper lungs. It is not the goal, when working with breathing exercises, to inhale as fully and forcefully as possible, but, rather, to *gently* fill the lungs, without strain, with prana, in the form of breath ... the sustaining force of life.

Retention - following ingestion (puraka), the breath is retained for a brief, but specific, count. This retention is called **antara-kumbhaka**. The breath is retained for various lengths of time following both inhalation and exhalation (**biya-kumbaka**), for several reasons: 1) at the physiological level, breath retention enables the system the time necessary to change and exchange in the lungs the gases (oxygen and carbon dioxide) in the blood; 2) retention of breath also helps the practitioner develop self discipline and, ultimately, control and focus of the mind. (Once again, we're using the work with the body to influence the mind!) Consciously working with controlled breathing, one exerts subtle and positive influences over most of the other systems of the body ... including digestion, circulation (blood pressure, pulse rate), and the endocrine (glandular) system.

Exhalation - **rechaka** - is also practiced in two stages: first, the diaphragm is drawn in, toward the spine, to expel the air gently from the base of the lungs; next, the chest muscles are relaxed to enable breath expulsion from the upper lungs.

Note: The breathing exercises of yoga thoroughly oxygenate the body ... including the brain; so some light-headedness may occur. This is due to the brain being unaccustomed to receiving an appropriate quantity of oxygen. When this occurs, simply discontinue the breathing exercise for several seconds or minutes, breathe gently and abdominally, then continue work with the chosen exercise. In time, and with practice, as the brain becomes accustomed to being properly oxygenated, unpleasant sensations associated with the breathing exercises will pass.

One who hates violence will not find peace, for only one who loves peace can know peace. We feel justified in our hatred because we believe we hate only that which is evil. But any hatred forms a strong bond, and in time we must realize it is hatred itself that is the destroyer.

Seth

PRANAYAMAS

The Breathing Technique of ...
Sukh Purvak ... The Rhythmic Breath

Yogic breathing, like life itself, is based on rhythm. The rhythmic ratio practiced in the breathing technique known as **Sukh Purvak** (1:4:2:1) is recommended. For instance, inhale to a count of 3, retain the breath for a count of 12, exhale to the count of 6, and hold the breath out for a count of 3 ... and repeat. Complete about six rounds of this exercise, then sit quietly for several minutes with the breathing gentle and *abdominal*. Body and mind systems will *naturally* begin to coordinate and harmonize. In time, one may want to increase the practice ratio to 4:16:8:4 or even to 5:20:10:5.

As previously mentioned, when one is inactive, and in a relaxed state, breathing should always be gentle and abdominal ... with just the diaphragm slowly expanding and relaxing ... no upper chest movement at all. In this way, the life force known as prana is gently drawn to the base of the lungs with each calm breath. The mind is quieted and the body is continuously oxygenated. Practice abdominal breathing whenever you think of it – when driving the car or sitting behind the desk or anytime the body is mostly inactive; in a fairly short period of time (usually weeks), abdominal breathing will become the body "norm" and you will no longer have to *think* about it. It will become *natural* breathing.

The technique:

1) Sit comfortably with the spine, neck, and head in alignment.

2) Relax the muscles of the chest and abdomen, enabling the release of all but the residual air from the lungs.

3) Begin the inhalation (puraka) by expanding just the abdomen. The rib cage remains immobile. Continue puraka (inhalation), now relaxing the diaphragm and expanding the rib cage to fully fill the lungs ... for your chosen ratio count.

4) Retain the breath (antara-kumbhaka) for your chosen ratio count. Keep the throat open; use the muscles of the chest to hold the breath in.

5) Begin the exhalation for the chosen count (rechaka) by first drawing the abdominal muscles in; complete rechaka by contracting the upper chest muscles ... finally tensing abdominal and chest muscles, and *squeezing* the breath thoroughly from the lungs.

6) Hold the breath out (biya-kumbaka) for the proper count.

Inhale (puraka) and repeat the exercise five to ten rounds. Practice focusing the awareness *just* on the breath during the exercise. As with all practices, let the focus of awareness be with *just this*. *Remember:* If you become lightheaded during the breathing exercises, you may want to limit the number of rounds ... but keep up the practice!

PRANAYAMAS

The Breathing Technique of ...
Nadi-Sadhana ... Alternate Nostril Breathing

Alternate Nostril Breathing helps establish stillness and calmness in mind and body, and prepares an environment conducive to sitting in meditation. Nadi is a Sanskrit word which is a general reference to energy channels, or, more physically-specific, to the nervous system of the body. Sadhana refers to any and all cleansing practices ... physiological, psychological, and spiritual. Western clinical studies have shown that continued breathing exclusively through one nostril has a measurable affect on the opposite hemisphere of the brain ... and stimulates the abilities and characteristics of that brain hemisphere.

The Sanskrit word Sushumna refers to the energy/nerve channel found in the body's spinal column ... the principle conduit of nerve energy in the body ... which extends from the base of the brain to the abdomen (to the Solar Plexus, or Sun Center). On either side of Sushumna are smaller nerve conduits called Ida (left) and Pingala (right).

The objective in working with breathing techniques is not simply to ingest prana (energy), but, more profoundly, to learn to *control* ... positively direct ... that energy. Therefore, it is important, when working with pranayamas, to utilize the power of visualization ... to *see* the flow of Nadi Sadhana. When breath is ingested through one nostril, *see* – visualize - it flow to the throat; at the throat visualize that energy of breath cross to the opposite side of Sushumna (the spine), and flow down that channel to the base of the spine ... resting in the abdomen - The Solar Plexus ... the Sun Center. When the breath is released on an exhalation (rechaka), *see* it flowing up the channel opposite the one it previously passed down, crossing again at the throat, and flowing out the opposite nostril. Reverse and repeat the process, inhaling through the opposite nostril ... and, again, visualizing the flow of breath-energy.

The Technique (suggested breathing ratio 1:4:2:1):

1) Sit comfortably with the spine, neck, and head in alignment. Place either hand so that the three middle fingers rest on the forehead, at a point just above and between the eyebrows (the ajna). The thumb and little finger rest on either side of the opposite nostrils ... facilitating (or inhibiting) the flow of breath through that nostril.

2) Exhale completely and evenly through both nostrils.

14

3) Press closed the left nostril. To your chosen count, inhale (puraka) through the right nostril. (Visualize the breath flowing through the right nostril, crossing at the throat, and flowing evenly down the Ida (left) channel to rest in the abdomen.) Retain the breath (kumbhaka) for your chosen count ... with the awareness focused on the breath resting in the abdomen.

4) Drawing the abdomen in, exhale (rechaka). Visualize the breath flowing up the opposite (Pingala - right) nerve channel, crossing at the throat, and flowing out the left nostril.

5) Hold the breath out (kumbhaka) for the chosen count. Inhale through the left nostril and repeat the process for the other nostril.

This completes one cycle. Practice three to five cycles initially ... five to ten cycles, eventually. If you become dizzy, limit the number of rounds until the brain adjusts to the increased oxygen flow, then increase the rounds to three to five per practice.

Following Nadi Sadhana, sit quietly and contemplatively in meditation for several minutes. Teach the mind to focus only on the gentle flow of breath into and out of the nostrils as the abdomen calmly expands and relaxes. Refer to the section of this book on the "Vipasana – Just Noticing" meditation technique to complement the practice of Nadi Sadhana.

PRANAYAMAS

The Breathing Technique of ...
Bastrika ... The Bellows Breath

Bastrika is a very invigorating, stimulating breathing exercise. The blood is quickly oxygenated, and the rapid movement of the exercise naturally stimulates the body's nervous system. However, the result is not "nervousness", as we might usually think of it ... quite the opposite. We experience a sensation of peace and calm, yet accompanied by a peaked sense of alertness and awareness.

Because of the rapid, snapping motion in the abdomen during the Bastrika exercise, it is advised that the stomach be empty and the nasal passages be very clean ... perhaps with tissue paper handy.

The technique:

1) Assume a comfortable sitting posture ... either cross-legged or Vajrasana (legs folded under). Completely relax the breathing until the movement in the abdomen is very slow and calm.

2) Exhale quickly, forcefully, sharply, and rapidly - by producing an inward snapping motion in the abdomen ... forcing the air out through the nostrils as you might when blowing your nose.

3) Rapidly expand the abdomen – not a complete upper-chest inhalation - but just enough to replace the expelled air. Without hesitation, snap the breath out again ... in again ... out again ... in again ... out again ... repeatedly ... continuously ... ten to twenty times.

4) Following ten to twenty repetitions of Bastrika, relax the breathing for a moment, allowing the breath to flow calmly and abdominally; then repeat the exercise two to three more rounds.

Following the work with Bastrika, take a long, slow, complete inhalation. Retain the breath for several seconds, then release it slowly and completely. Sit with relaxed breathing for two or three minutes; let the mind just casually observe the body's sense-sations.

PRANAYAMAS

The Breathing Technique of ...
Agni-sara Dhati ...The Fire Breath

Agni means "fire" in Sanskrit, and Agni-sara Dhati is referred to as The Fire Breath. It is a vigorous, abdominal breathing technique that stimulates digestion and develops and tones the abdominal muscles. It is suggested that the nasal passages be clean and open, and the stomach empty, when practicing this exercise.

The technique:

1) Assume a comfortable sitting posture ... either cross-legged or in Vajrasana (legs folded under). Completely relax the breathing until the movement in the abdomen becomes slow and calm.

2) Exhale forcefully ... not sharp and rapidly, as in Bastrika, but simply and vigorously drawing the abdomen in as completely as possible. Visualize as if your objective is to draw the stomach muscles all the way to touching the lower spine. Hesitate for one or two seconds, then ...

3) Inhale slowly, but vigorously and forcefully, just into the abdomen ... expanding the stomach as completely as possible. There should be no upper-chest movement at all, just the stomach expanding like a rapidly-filled balloon. Hesitate for one or two seconds, then ...

4) Exhale forcefully again ... as in step #2 above.

5) Continue to breathe vigorously into and out of the abdomen, completing eight to ten rounds of Agni-sara Dhati. Then relax the breathing once again ... let the breath become gentle and abdominal, restful and meditative. Feel and visualize the warm glow, the "fire", radiating from the solar plexus.

Remember: the breathing exercises of yoga thoroughly oxygenate the body ... including the brain; so some light-headedness may occur. This is due to the brain not being accustomed to receiving appropriate oxygen. When this occurs, simply discontinue the breathing exercise for several seconds or minutes, breathe gently and abdominally, then continue work with the specific exercise. In time, and with practice, as the brain becomes accustomed to being properly oxygenated, the unpleasant sensations associated with the breathing exercises will pass.

Basic Standing Postures

Our standing routine includes work with a variety of asanas that stretch the body forward and back, and twist from side to side. First …

Bring the body to a standing posture … feeling the change and feeling the movement. Rest the body in its standing posture. Simply *feel* the body standing. Feel the soles of the feet pressed against the floor. Feel the arms hanging limp and relaxed at the sides … so relaxed you can even feel the gentle pulsing sensation in the fingertips. Take a moment to just focus the awareness on standing. Then …

PADAHASTASANA

Standing Head-to-Knee

Padahastasana, the standing head-to-knee pose, combines many of the benefits of Pashimatana (the sitting head-to-knee pose) with the simple inversion postures. By reversing the effects of gravity, from the heart up, on the body's circulation system, the brain and the glands and organs in the head are cleansed and rejuvenated; the posterior muscles are vigorously stretched, and the sense of physical balance (crucial to the development of a centered mind) is greatly enhanced.

1) Stand relaxed with the spine, head, and neck in alignment, and the shoulders back. Let the body's weight rest evenly over the soles of the feet, and take a moment to focus the awareness on the body in its standing posture … observing the various sense-sations. Exhale completely and then inhale slowly and completely. Let the head drop back, vigorously stretching the neck. As you exhale …

2) Bend forward from the waist and slide the hands down the back of the legs pressing the palms against the calves, using the leverage in the arms to pull the upper body gently toward the legs.

3) Apply gentle stretch … not enough to feel strain. Relax the breathing and hold the posture for 30 seconds to a minute. Exhale completely, and as you inhale …

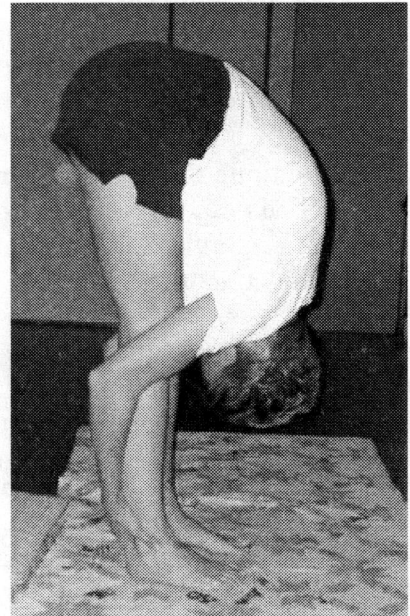

18

4) *Gradually* curl the body up ... pulling the body slowly from the base of the spine back to an upright position.

5) Place the hands at the lower back, exhale and arch the body vigorously. Inhale and s-l-o-w-l-y straighten the spine. Relax the breathing; briefly re-center before continuing with the next asana.

Take a moment to re-center the mind, bring the breath back to slow and abdominal, and rest.

TRIKONASANA

The Triangle Pose

Trikonasana complements and combines the benefits of a simple, gentle body twist with a partial inversion, and a vigorous posterior stretch.

Version one -

1) Stand with the feet about a yard apart. Exhale completely. As you inhale ...

2) Extend the straightened arms, palms down, perpendicular to the body and parallel to the floor. As you exhale ...

3) Twist the body to the right (or either side), simultaneously bend forward from the waist, and bring the left hand to the top of the right foot (or resting on the right shin, depending on hamstring flexibility; try not to bend the knees). Extend the right arm straight up toward the ceiling, and twist the head to gaze up toward the ceiling.

4) Relax the breathing. Hold the posture for 30 seconds to a minute. Increase the length of time (up to 2 minutes) with practice. Exhale completely, and as you inhale ...

5) Release the posture by pulling the body upright from the waist, but keep the arms extended and maintain the twist to the right. Exhale, swivel the body to the left and duplicate the reverse of the procedure on the other side.

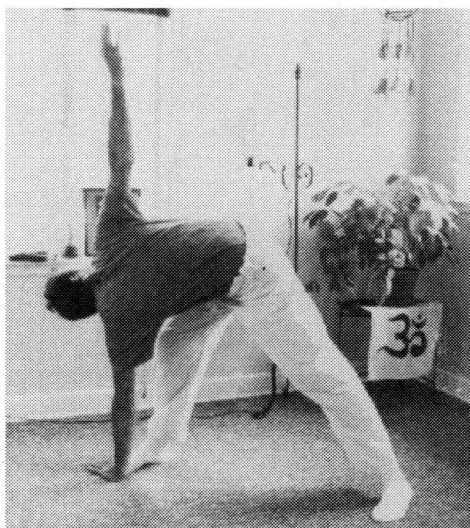

Version two –

1) With the feet still about a yard apart, and the arms still extended perpendicular to the body and parallel to the floor, take a deep and complete inhalation. As you exhale ...

2) Bend/lean the body to the right (or either side), placing the right hand to the side of the right leg ... still facing forward ... and bringing the left arm and the upper torso as parallel to the floor as possible.

3) Hold the posture for 30 seconds to a minute (eventually to two minutes, if possible). Exhale completely and focus the awareness to the base of the stretching side. Then, as you inhale ...

4) Pull the body upright from that point ... pull the body up from the base of the stretching side ... slowly and consciously.

5) Reverse, and stretch the other side.

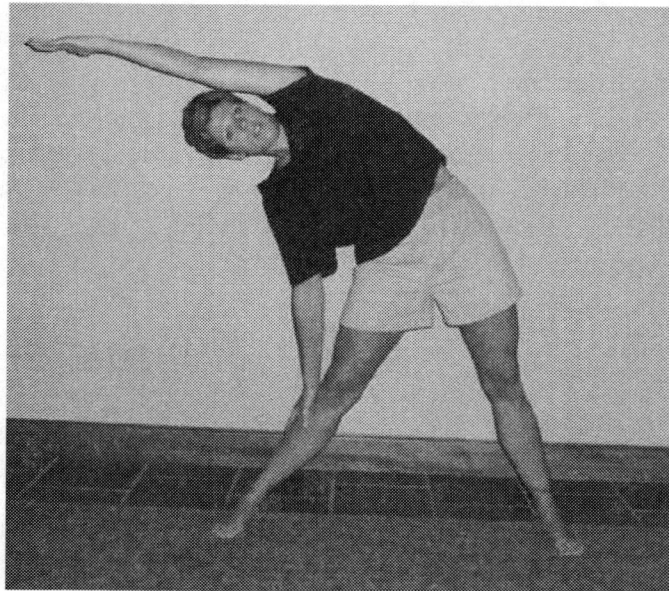

The lesson which life repeats and constantly re-enforces is this: "Look under foot!" We are always nearer The Divine and The True Sources of our power than we think. The lure of the distant, the difficult, and the exotic is deceptive. The great opportunity is where we are ... now ... in the moment. So, do not despise your own place and hour, for every place is under the stars and every place is the center of the universe.

John Burroughs

VRIKSHANA

The Tree Pose

The word "coordination" literally means to be with (co) a point (ordinate) or, in a specific psycho/physical place. Thus, in Yoga, "coordination" means to be with one-pointedness. The Tree Pose, Vrikshasana, is a standing balancing posture which helps one develop co-ordination... one-pointedness with mind, breath, and body; and helps the student learn to flow with the forces of nature, rather than be in opposition to them.

1) Stand straight, but not too rigid. Lean slightly to the left or right ... until the body's weight is aligned comfortably over that leg.

2) Bend the other knee, positioning that foot high to the inside of the straightened thigh ... toes pointing down. Extend the arms, as necessary, to maintain balance.

3) While balancing on one foot, slowly raise the arms overhead until the palms join. Breathe slowly and diaphragmatically. Let the eyes gaze steadily on a neutral focal point. Feel the balance ... as effortlessly as possible. If and when balance is lost, simply resume work with the asana. Be absolutely unconcerned with success or failure. Hold the posture for 30 seconds to, if possible, one full minute.

4) Release the posture on an exhalation, bringing the arms down in a wide lateral sweeping motion, and lowering the raised foot back to the floor.

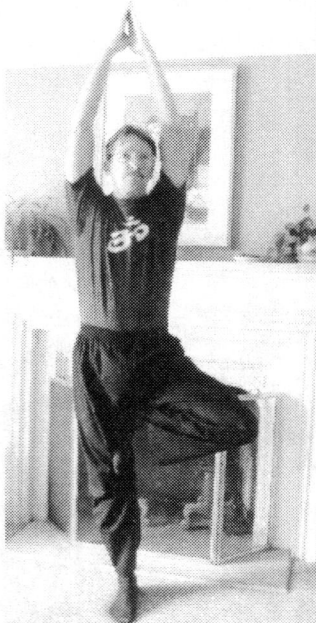

5) Repeat on the other side.

Practicing balancing postures enables learning passive concentration ... *effortless* effort. When resting in passive awareness, the student experiences what Zen yogis call: satori. Satori occurs when the mind is free of thought, yet fully aware; the body is alert and sensitive, yet completely relaxed. The mind is not trapped by emotions.

THREE VIGOROUS BREATHS

This simple exercise vigorously stimulates and invigorates both body and mind, while stretching the muscles and enhancing one's balancing practice ...

1) Rest the body in a standing posture, facing forward, with both arms relaxed at the sides ... head, neck, and spine in comfortable alignment.

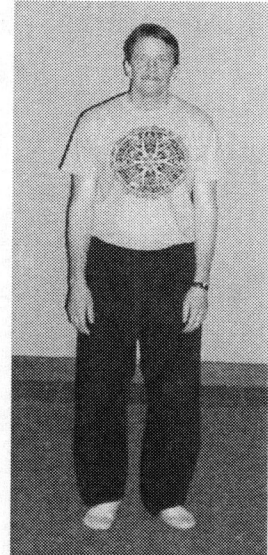

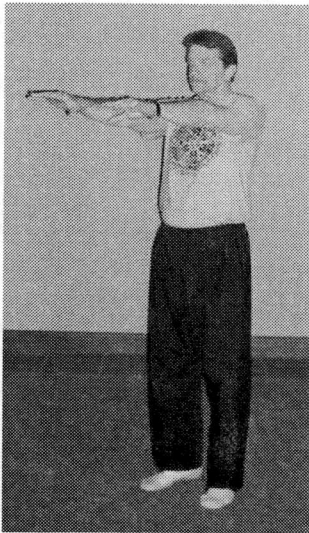

2) Exhale slowly, completely, and consciously. Then rapidly and vigorously inhale, through the nostrils, into the lower third of the lungs (expanding the abdomen). Simultaneously extend the arms before you, perpendicular to the front of the body. Briefly pause, then ...

3) ... rapidly and vigorously inhale into the middle third of the lungs (relaxing the abdominal muscles). Simultaneously and rapidly swing and extend the arms straight out from the body. Briefly pause, then ...

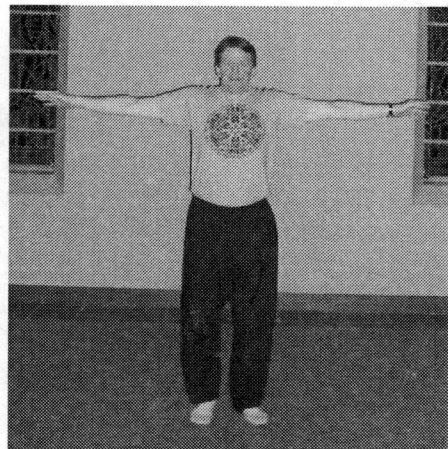

4) … rapidly and vigorously inhale into the upper third of the lungs (expanding the chest while drawing the abdomen in). Simultaneously extend the arms directly overhead, palms together and touching. Lift the body up, onto the toes, stretching with vigor, and balancing. Briefly pause, then …

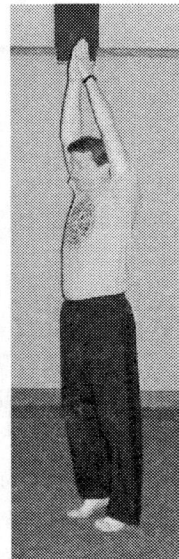

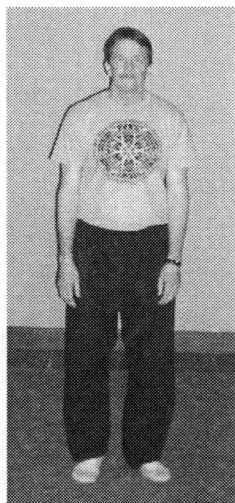

5) … retaining the breath, on a slow, continuous exhalation (first drawing the abdomen in) lower the feet back to the floor and, as the breath is released, simultaneously lower the hands and arms down the front of the body (in alignment with Sushumna … the spine), bringing the arms back to a position adjacent to the sides. Take a deep, complete inhalation, exhale, and …

6) Repeat twice more.

*Then I was standing on the highest mountain of them all, and 'round about beneath me was the whole hoop of the world. And while I stood there I saw more than I can tell, and I understood more than I saw; for I was seeing in a sacred manner the shapes of all things of the spirit, and the shape of all shapes as they must live together as one being. And I saw that the sacred hoop of my people was one of many hoops that all make but One Circle ... wide as the daylight and the starlight, and in the center of that circle grew a mighty, flowering tree! A tree to shelter **all** of the children ... children of the one Mother and of the one Father. And I saw that it was Holy.*

Black Elk

Suggested Beginner's
Hatha Yoga Routine

The beginning student may wish to work with the following routine for 30 minutes to an hour daily, as meets *your* specific needs and requirements -

I)   Sit and Center - Focus the awareness on the gentle, abdominal breath for two or three minutes before beginning work with the asanas (postures).

II) Stretch the body in sitting postures: Pashimatana (head-to-knee; both legs straight) and Bhodi-konasana (The Butterfly). *Move* into the postures slowly and *consciously*, holding the postures for one to two minutes.

III) Stand and Center - Focus the awareness on the sensations of the body while simply standing balanced (Tadasana) for two or three minutes, then ...

IV) Stretch the body in Padahastasana (standing head-to-knee), then Trikonasana (Triangle). Balance and center body and mind with Vrikshasana (Tree Pose).

V)   Reassume a sitting posture. Sit quietly for three or four minutes while practicing focusing the awareness *totally* on the breath. Complete six rounds of Sukh Purvak (rhythmic breath), followed by Janu-sirasana (head-to-knee; one leg bent). Complete the sitting work with a round of Neck Exercises.

VI) Exhale the body to a back-reclining posture and vigorously arch the spine two or three times. Then stimulate and increase overall strength with five rounds of the Swiss Movement (see page 39). Relax *consciously* in Savasana for ten to fifteen minutes.

Note: This routine is just a *suggestion*. Feel free to modify it (add or delete specific asanas), or change the order and/or length of time postures are held, as your practice progresses and you begin to identify your personal needs.

SURYA NAMASKAR

The Sun Salutation

Surya Namaskar combines several yoga asanas into a series of graceful, flowing movements. The movements may be executed rapidly, creating an aerobic affect, or slowly, emphasizing each individual posture – or even holding each posture for several seconds or minutes, working with them as asanas. Regardless of the pace, Surya Namaskar should always be practiced with grace, and with awareness focused on the execution of the movements. Crucial to proper practice is co-ordination of movement and breath. Inhalations, exhalations, and breath retention all flow in harmony with the changes in body positioning. Surya Namaskar is an excellent prelude to calming and resting the body in Savasana (Deep Relaxation). Refer to the series of illustrations below ...

1) Stand straight, but relaxed, with the feet within a couple of inches of one another. Place the palms of the hands together before the heart ... in the traditional prayer posture. Exhale consciously and completely. As you inhale ...

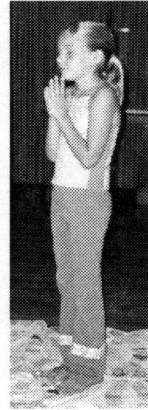

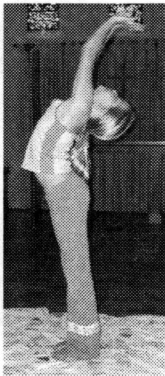

2) Straighten and lift the arms up and overhead, and arch the back vigorously.

As you exhale ...

3) Bend forward from the waist, bringing the hands to rest adjacent to each foot. (Note: If flexibility does not enable touching the floor, simply extend the arms parallel to the legs and point the fingers toward the floor.) Keep the legs straight. The body is now in a modified version of Padahastasana (standing head-to-knee posture). As you inhale ...

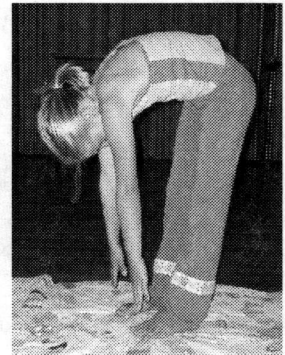

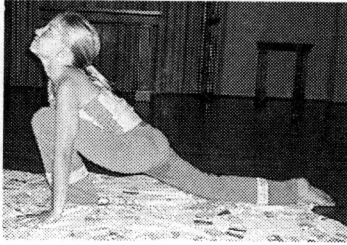

4) Extend the right leg straight back, with the toes curled under, and either lower the knee to the floor for support, or keep the extended right leg straight ... as you choose. Hands remain in place. Lift the head up and back as far as possible. This posture is called Ardha-Bhujangasana - the Half-Cobra pose. Retain the breath and ...

5) Straighten the left leg parallel to the right ... supporting the body in the traditional push-up posture. As you exhale ..

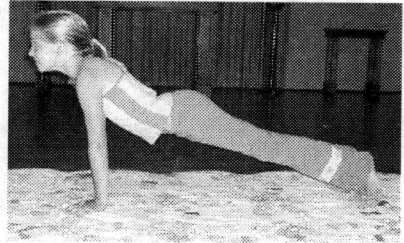

6) Lower the body to the floor ... to the 8-pointed posture: the forehead, knees, and chest touch the floor, while the lower back is sharply arched and the pelvis and buttocks are slightly elevated off the floor. After holding the 8-pointed posture for a moment, flatten the body on the floor and on an inhalation ...

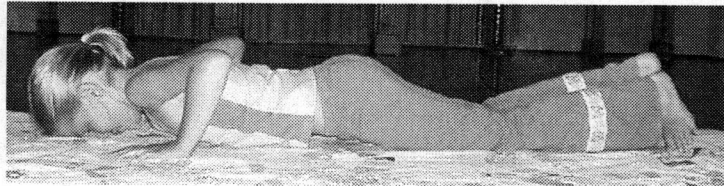

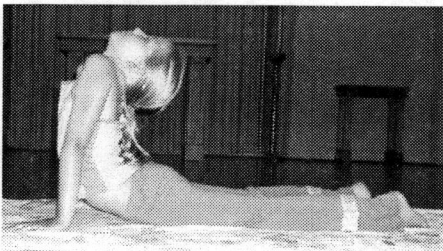

7) Arch to Bhujangasana ... the Cobra pose. Curl the toes under, and as you exhale ...

8) Lift the body to form an inverted "V". Bring the feet forward a few inches, if necessary, elevate the hips high and press down vigorously on the heels. Allow the head to hang limp and at rest. (Variation: While holding the inverted-V, inhale and lift the head up and back as far as is comfortably possible; lower the head on an exhalation.) As you inhale ...

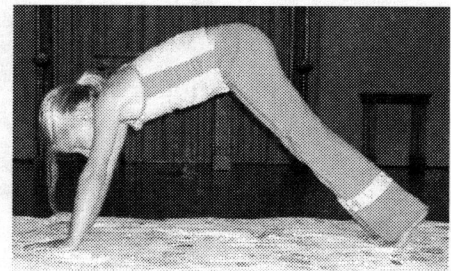

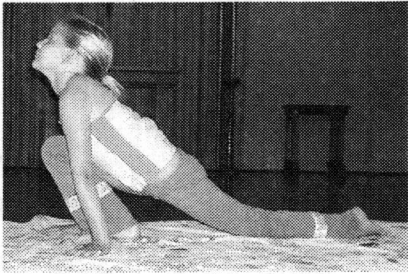

9) Bring the right foot forward, reversing the positioning of the legs (described in #4, above) ... once again assuming Ardha-Bhujangasana (Half Cobra). On an exhalation ...

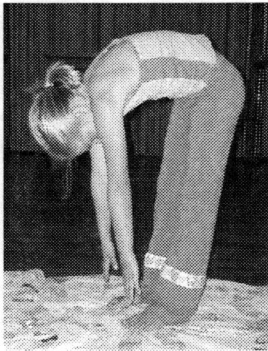

10) Bring the left foot forward, lifting the body once again to the Standing Head-to-Knee posture (Padahastasana ... as in #3, above). Inhale deeply, and ...

11) Slowly curl the spine up and straight as you lift the arms up and overhead, and arch the back vigorously. Exhale and reassume the prayer posture ... or, if continuing the movements, exhale back to the Standing Head-to-Knee pose.

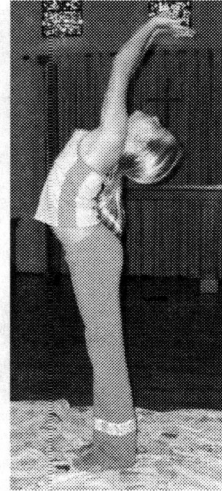

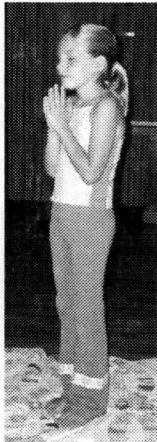

Four to six rounds of Surya Namaskar are generally considered sufficient. You may want to hold the various postures, during one of those rounds, to combine the work of asana with exercise.

A note on the prayer posture (with which we begin and conclude this series of movements): The prayer posture, or "Namaste posture" as it is sometimes called, symbolizes the two coming together as one. Although the hands are still "individual", they are no longer separate. So it is with yoga: the worldly self *joins* with the spiritual self. This joining, uniting, linking together of all of the aspects of our being is what the word "yoga" means. Yoga means "union". As beings, we retain our individuality … but not our sense of separateness.

The illustration below shows the complete series of Surya Namaskar movements. This exercise may be practiced rapidly – aerobically, or slowly and meditatively, or the various postures can each be held at length as you flow through the series of movements.

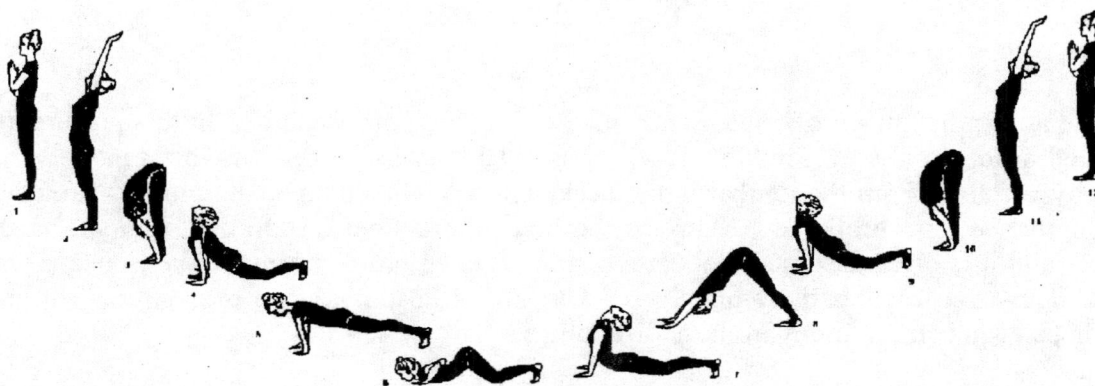

The twelve steps of Surya Namaskar

Reclining Stomach Exercises

The following exercises and asanas are performed while lying in a reclining position on the stomach. With creative yogic thinking, the practitioner can, and should, execute the asanas as a moving meditation … with graceful, flowing motions … so that the practice becomes, not just exercises for the body, but also a focal point for the mind.

BHUJANGASANA

The Cobra Pose

In the ancient language of yoga, Sanskrit, "Bhujanga" means "cobra". In this posture, the arched head and body resemble an alert cobra. Bhujangasana benefits the spine … vertebra by vertebra, from the lumbar to the neck. The spinal column (sushumna) is stretched, strengthened, and limbered. Many of the body's structural difficulties originate in the back, and it is often assumed that certain spine-related problems unavoidably occur with age. However, regular daily practice of The Cobra Pose is said to prevent, and in time perhaps even correct, many of these difficulties.

Note: If you are currently experiencing back problems, the Cobra Pose (as with all of the postures, all of the time) should be practiced *gently and cautiously*. Most structural problems develop over a period of years and must be corrected gradually. Thus, practice should always be gentle … but regular and consistent.

1) Lie flat on the stomach, face down, chin touching chest, and the forehead resting on the floor. Extend the arms parallel to the body, palms up. Exhale completely and relax all muscles. As you inhale ...

2) Slowly lift the head and begin arching the shoulders and upper spine. Simultaneously bring the hands forward and place them, palms down, adjacent to the shoulders.

3) Continue the inhalation. With the strength in the arms, slowly raise the body and arch the spine until the navel is slightly off the floor.

Variation: If the spine is too stiff and inflexible for the full posture, support the body with the *forearms* flat on the floor, while still arching as vigorously as possible … without strain.

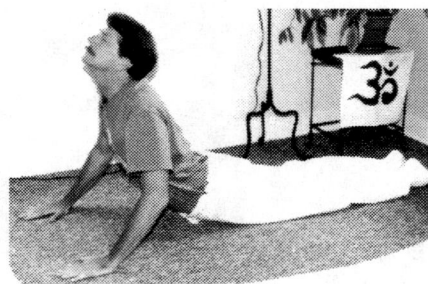

4) Relax the breathing (abdominal breath) and hold the posture for 15 to 30 seconds, initially ... 1 to 2 minutes, eventually. Exhale ...

5) Release the posture and reverse the initial movements, lowering the body back to the floor. As the spine unfurls, continue to hold the shoulders and head back; *then*, lower the shoulders to the floor; *then*, lower the head back to its starting position.

An important concept in yoga is balance. Postures should be followed by counter-balancing movements or poses. Therefore, the backward-bending spine-flexing vigorous Bhujangasana should be balanced with ...

BALASANA

The Fallen Leaf Posture

1) Following the release of The Cobra Pose, and while resting in its starting position, place the hands adjacent to the shoulders and begin to arch the body off the floor ... as if assuming Bhujangasana, but ...

2) Lift the body up onto the knees and fold the body back so that the torso rests folded on the thighs, and the forehead rests on the floor. Extend the arms either before you, or adjacent to the sides, or place the hands one over the other and rest the forehead on the back of the hands.

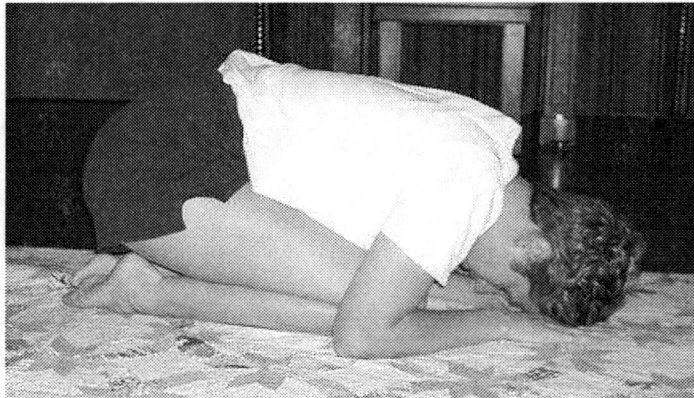

After resting in this posture for about one full minute, *very slowly* (meditatively!), on an inhalation, curl the body to the Vajrasana (Diamond Pose) sitting position. Feel and visualize as each vertebra aligns one atop the other. Once in Vajrasana, place your hands behind you, palms flat on the floor, and arch vigorously. Sit in The Diamond Pose, resting the breath, for about a minute; then, consciously continue with your practice ...

ARDHA – SALABASANA
and SALABASANA

The Half & Full Locust

Ardha-Salabasana and Salabasana strengthen and flex the lower back and leg muscles, and gently realign the pelvic and spinal regions of the skeletal system. The Salabasanas (both half & full), while strengthening the lower back, complement many of the benefits of Bhujangasana, the Cobra Pose. While the Cobra more directly affects the upper body (stretching the chest and abdominal muscles and strengthening the arms and shoulders), the Salabasanas specifically affect the lower body.

Ardha (Half) - Salabasana (Locust):

1) Lie flat on the stomach with the chin resting on the floor, and the arms extended adjacent to the body, palms down, elbows slightly bent. Exhale completely, consciously releasing all tension from the body. As you inhale deeply ...

2) Lift the straightened right leg from the floor as high as comfortably possible, without rolling the body to the side. Support and steady the body with hands and arms. Retain the breath and the posture for about 10 to 15 seconds. Lower the leg back to its starting position on a slow, gentle exhalation. As you inhale fully again ...

3) Lift the straightened left leg off the floor as high as comfortably possible. Again, use the hands to support and steady the body, and retain the breath and posture for about 10 to 15 seconds. Lower the leg back to its starting position on a slow, gentle exhalation. Repeat with each leg.

Salabasana (Full Locust):

4) On a deep inhalation, lift both legs from the floor as high as comfortably possible, press down firmly with the hands and arms. Retain the breath and the posture for 5 to 10 seconds. Slowly lower the legs back to the floor on an exhalation.

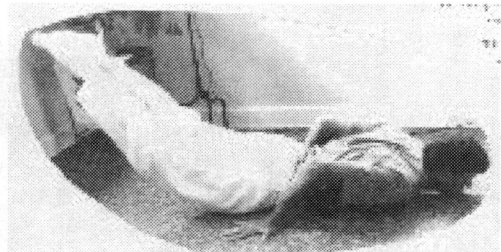

6) Rest in the Fallen Leaf posture for about a minute, then, on a *slow* inhalation, curl the body upright to the Vajrasana sitting posture. Place your hands behind you flat on the floor and, as you exhale, arch the spine vigorously. Release.

DHANURASANA

The Bow Pose

Dhanurasana, the Bow pose, offers many of the same benefits as other back-flexing and chest-stretching exercises, such as Bhujangasana (the Cobra) and Ustrasana (the Camel). However, the Bow pose is more vigorous than the Camel and Cobra postures, and unlike some other back-bending postures also works with the skeletal structure in the legs ... especially the knees. The Bow Pose is also isometric and helps to develop and maintain leg and arm muscles.

1) Begin lying on the stomach with the chin resting on the floor. Bend the knees, placing the tops of the feet in the hands, or grasp the ankles. Keep the knees as close together as is comfortably possible. Exhale completely. As you inhale ...

2) Lift the head up and back and arch the spine as vigorously as possible. Keep the head back, stretching the throat, and simultaneously pull against the feet with the hands and push against the hands with the feet. Breathe gently and hold the posture for fifteen to thirty seconds. Then, inhale and arch as vigorously as possible, and on an exhalation ...

3) Lower the chest and head back to the floor, but maintain the grasp on the feet. Let the upper body rest on the floor and inhale deeply. Hold the breath and pull the feet in as close to the backs of the thighs as possible. As you exhale, retain the grasp on the feet, but release the vigorous pressure. Then, on an inhalation ...

4) Lift the head up and back ... again arching the body to the Bow Pose. Repeat steps two and three; complete two to four rounds of the asana.

5) Following the work with Dhanurasana, rest the body in Balasana ... The Fallen Leaf posture.

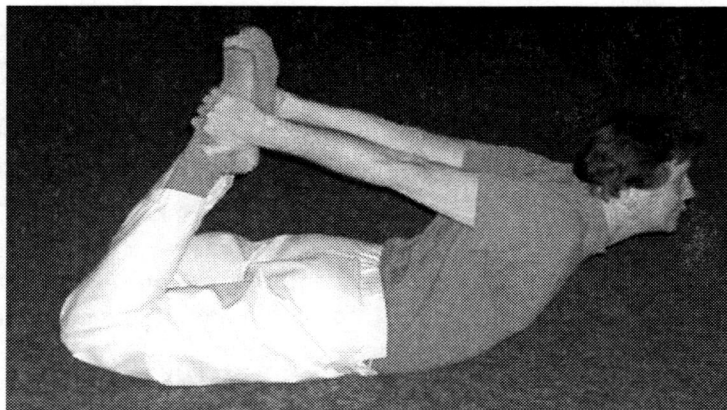

CAT STRETCH

Lower-back Exercise

This series of movements stretches the frontal muscles of the body ... from the feet to the throat. The lower back is strengthened and the body, although in a horizontal position, is vertically aligned.

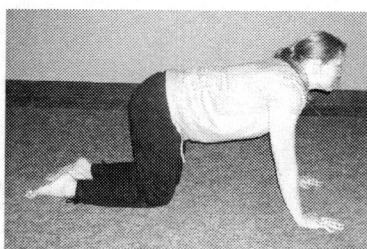

1) Begin with the body on the hands and knees, head facing gently forward. As always, begin working with the exercise with a full and complete exhalation, drawing the abdomen vigorously in. As you inhale

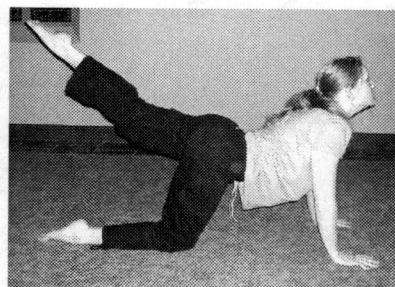

2) Straighten one leg and, keeping it straight, lift it as high as is comfortably possible. Lift the head up and back, stretching the throat vigorously. Retain the breath and hold the leg up and the head back for several seconds. On an exhalation ...

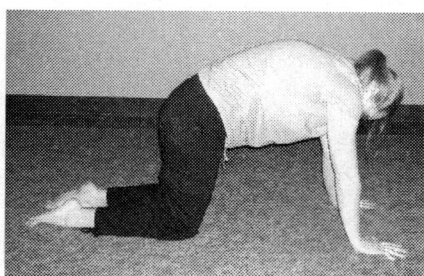

3) Lower the leg and head simultaneously, dropping the head down ... chin towards the chest. As the exhalation is completed, draw the stomach in vigorously, squeezing the air from the lungs, and arch the spine up as high as possible. Release, and as you inhale ...

4) Straighten the other leg, keeping it straight, lifting it as high as is comfortably possible. Lift the head up and back, stretching the throat vigorously. Retain the breath and hold the leg up and the head back for several seconds. On an exhalation ...

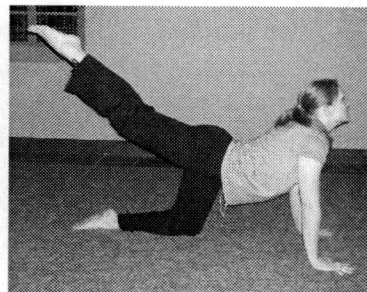

5) Lower that leg and the head simultaneously, dropping the head forward, chin to chest. As the exhalation is completed, draw the stomach in vigorously, squeezing the air from the lungs, and arch the spine up as high as possible. Release, and as you inhale …

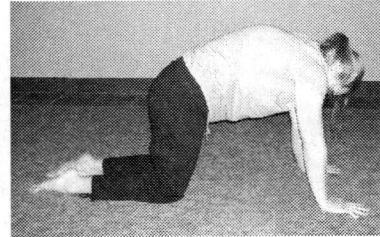

6) Repeat the movements two or three more times with each leg. Remember to move slowly and conscientiously … *meditatively* … with full awareness on what you are doing; visualize the body as you move it.

7) When you complete the final series, after exhaling vigorously and drawing the stomach muscles in firmly once again, as you inhale …

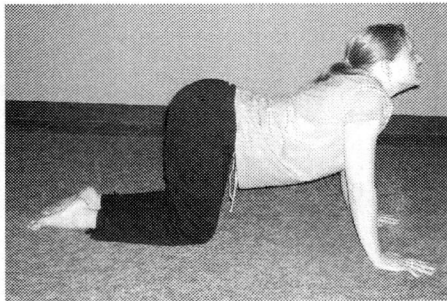

8) Press down with the lower back muscles as completely as possible, elevate the tailbone, and lift the head up and back. Press down vigorously (but not strenuously!) with the lower back muscles, stretch the throat vigorously, hold the posture for a few seconds. Release, and as you exhale …

9) Fold the body to the Fallen Leaf posture (Balasana) and rest for a few moments.

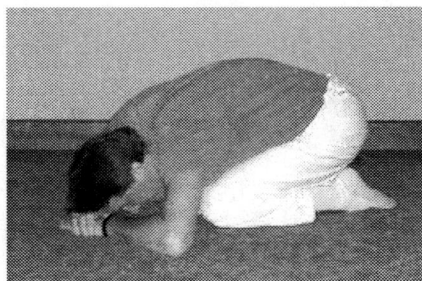

For the body does not consist only of one member, but of many. If the foot should say, "Because I am not a hand, I do not belong to the body," that would not make it any less a part of the body. And if the ear should say, "Because I am not an eye, I do not belong to the body," that would not make it any less a part of the body. For if the whole body were an eye, where would be the hearing? And if the whole body were an ear, where would be the feeling? But as it is, the organs are arranged in the body … each one of them according to purpose …

Corinthians

S A V A S A N A

Deep Relaxation

It has already been emphasized that relaxation is the essence of a yoga practice. Relaxing into the postures, and *with* the postures, teaches us how to relax with all that the day has to offer ... including, and especially, those experiences that are not to our liking. However, relaxation is a process and a specific technique, as well as a frame of mind. Concluding a yoga practice, or at any time we feel the need, we can practice the technique called Savasana. Savasana is ten- to twenty-minute deep relaxation practice. In addition to simply being pleasant, Savasana enables the body to assimilate the benefits and effects of exercises ... be they yoga, aerobic, or muscle/mass-building exercises ... and *enables* tensions and stress to be released.

The Technique:

1) Sit with the knees bent and the feet flat on the floor. Exhale completely, then take a deep and complete breath. As you exhale ...

2) S-l-o-w-l-y curl the spine down until the head rests on the floor. Then s-l-o-w-l-y straighten the legs and extend the arms adjacent to the sides with the palms up.

3) Breathing should be slow, gentle, and diaphragmatic ... the awareness should rest with the soothing rise and fall of the abdomen.

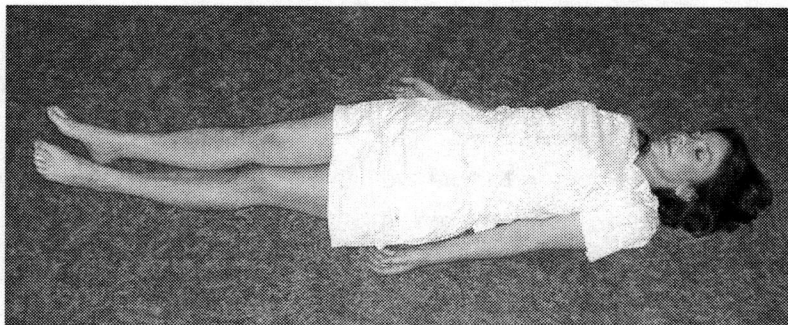

4) Exhale and vigorously tense the muscles of the legs; maintain the tension for several seconds, then release the tension suddenly, and as you inhale deeply *visualize* relaxation being drawn into the legs through the soles of the feet ... as if breathing directly into the legs. Slowly move the awareness up the body and ...

5) Systematically apply the same exhale/tensing and inhale/releasing technique to the pelvic area, the torso, the arms and hands. After clenching the fists and tensing the muscles of the arms, just as with the legs, release the tension suddenly and then inhale deeply and completely ... *visualizing* as if breathing directly into/through the palms of the hands and filling the arms with breath.

6) Finally, bring the awareness to the head. Squint the eyes and clench the teeth, as you exhale, and hold the facial muscles tense and tight. Release suddenly and inhale deeply, visualizing as if drawing the breath directly into/through the crown of the head ... as if filling the head with breath.

7) Now bring the awareness back to the gentle flow of breath in the nostrils, and to the soothing rise and fall of the abdomen.

8) Rest in Savasana for ten to twenty minutes. (It may be useful to set a timer.) If the mind drifts or wanders back to the concerns of the day, simply, and continuously, bring its focus back to the calming abdominal movement.

9) After resting in Savasana, consciously bend the knees and place the feet flat on the floor. Exhale completely. Inhale deeply and completely ... feel the body fill with fresh, invigorating air! ... and curl the body from the floor back to a sitting position. Sit for a few minutes, allowing time for the mind and body to regain full alertness.

We *consciously* practice the relaxation exercises of yoga so that we can experience the sensations of relaxation. Then, as we reenter the everyday world, remembering that experience, we begin to find we can practice those methods even as the day's events unfold. We can turn the awareness to the gentle abdominal breath at practically any time and bring a sense of rest and calm and *control* to situations that had previously seemed chaotic and beyond our influence.

Reclining Back Exercises

The following exercises and asanas are performed while lying in a reclining position on the back. The postures and exercises are designed primarily to develop back strength and flexibility, and also to invert the body ... to reverse the body's usual gravitational relationship ... and enable a fresh flow of blood to the brain and the organs of the head ... assisted by gravity now, rather than inhibited by it.

THE SWISS MOVEMENT

An Abdominal-strengthening Exercise

THE SWISS MOVEMENT is an active *exercise* (rather than a posture or asana) which strengthens the lower back and stomach muscles. Additionally, The Swiss Movement encourages deep, invigorating breathing and coordination of breath with bodily movement.

1) Lie flat on the back (as in Savasana ...the Relaxation posture); arms extended alongside the body, palms down. Exhale slowly and completely, relaxing all muscles in the body. As you inhale deeply, simultaneously ...

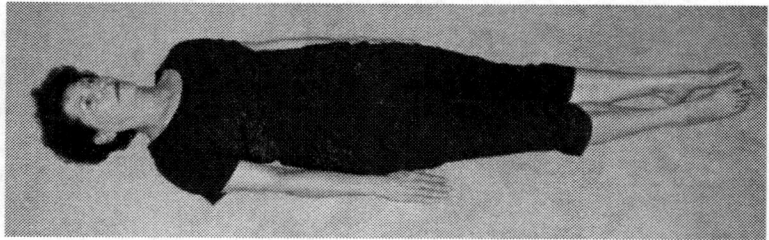

2) Lift the arms up and overhead to the floor.

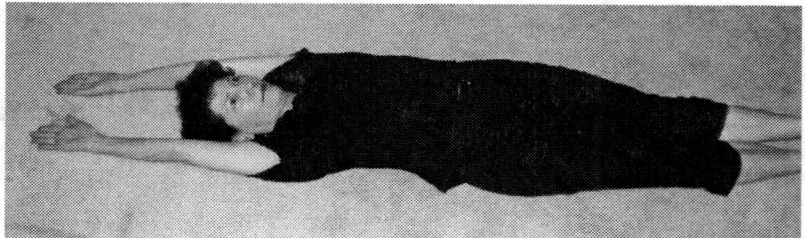

3) Exhale vigorously and rapidly through the mouth, and simultaneously bend the knees, folding the legs over the chest and wrapping the arms around the shins. Compress the legs tightly to the body. Inhale deeply and ...

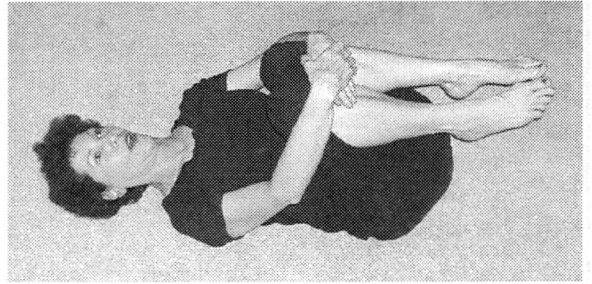

4) Straighten and extend the arms and legs toward the ceiling. While retaining the deep inhalation (or, while exhaling slowly, if you have high or low blood pressure) ...

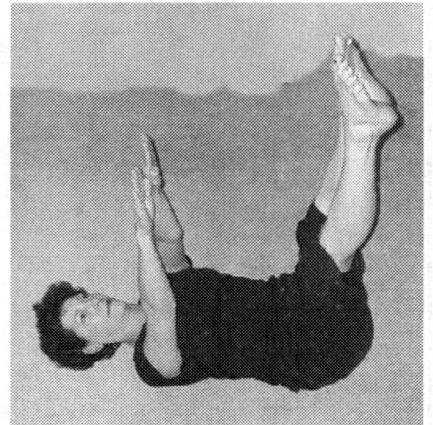

5) Simultaneously and slowly lower the straightened arms and legs back to the floor. Then, on a slow exhalation ...

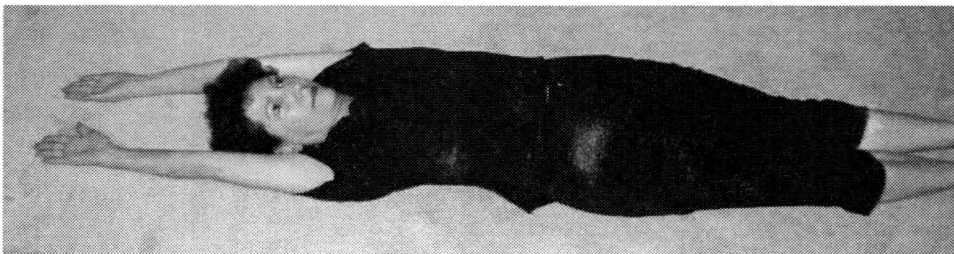

6) Lift the arms from the floor, swiveling them back to their starting position.

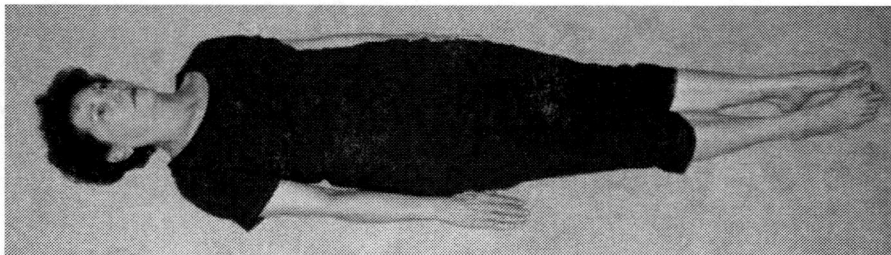

Repeat the exercise three to five times, then rest for a moment in Savasana.

LOWER BACK STRETCH

This series of simple stretches bring strength and flexibility to the lower back, and stretch the Achilles tendons.

1) Recline on the back, as in Savasana (the relaxation pose), but with the hands palms-down, the knees bent, and the feet flat on the floor. Exhale slowly and consciously, then take a deep, complete inhalation. As you exhale ...

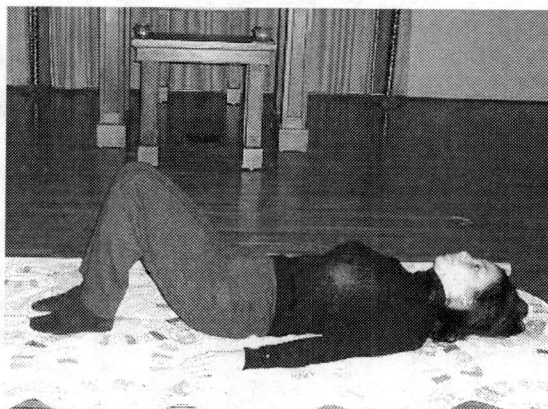

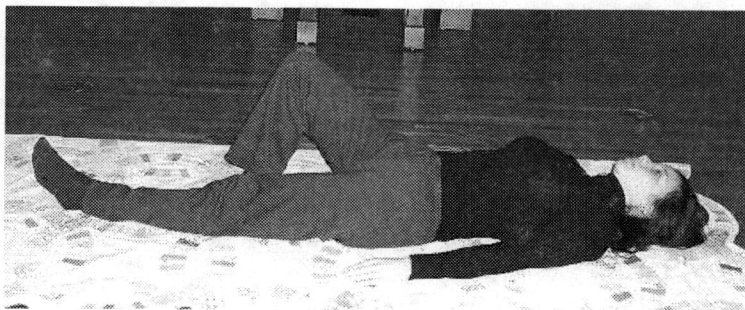

2) Slide one foot away, straightening that leg. Then, on an inhalation ...

3) Lift the straight leg off of the floor, bringing it as perpendicular to the body, or as towards the head, as is comfortably possible. Let the toes of the raised leg point down to the floor and press the heel toward the ceiling. Wrap the hands around the straightened leg, using the leverage in the arms to pull the leg gently forward.

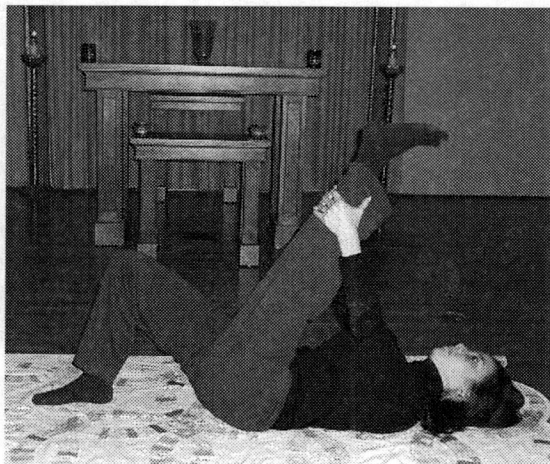

4) Hold the vigorous stretch for thirty seconds initially … a minute eventually … continuing to press the heel towards the ceiling and pull the leg forward. After holding the posture an appropriate length of time, exhale slowly and completely, then take a deep, complete breath. As you exhale …

5) Lower the leg slowly back to the floor. As you inhale …

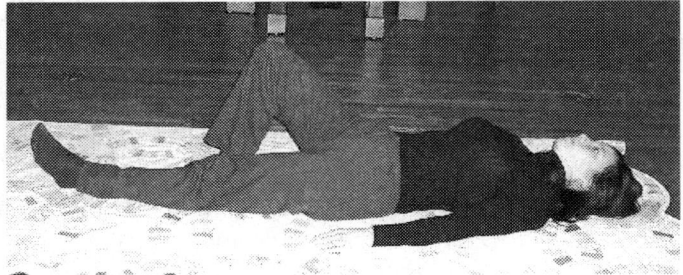

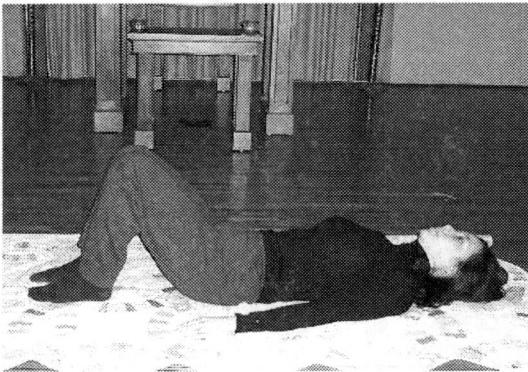

6) Bend the knee of the leg just stretched, bringing that foot back parallel to the other. Then, as you exhale …

7) Straighten the other leg. On an inhalation, repeat steps 3), 4), and 5) with that leg. After the second leg is returned to its starting position, take a deep inhalation, and as you exhale …

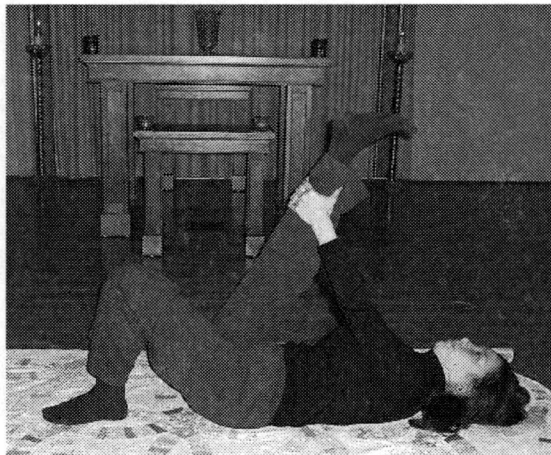

8) Slide the foot of the first leg away again ... so that both legs are now straight and side-by-side, with the feet relaxed but gently touching. Take a deep complete inhalation ...

9) And lift both feet just barely (an inch or two) off of the floor. Hold the breath, with the feet off the floor, for five to ten seconds. Release on an exhalation. Repeat step 9) two or three times.

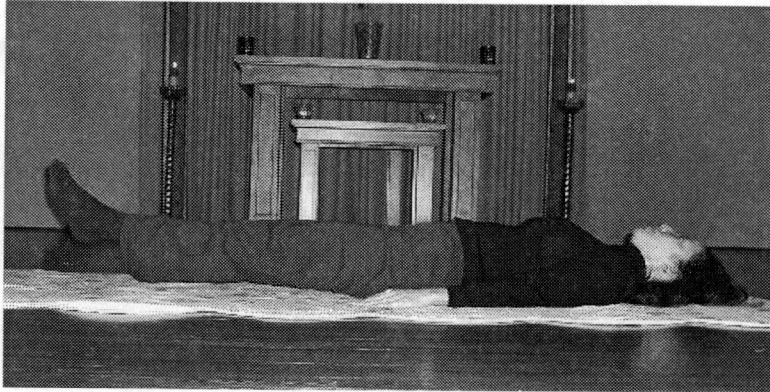

Suggestion: Following the individual work with both legs, you may wish to substitute step 9), or supplement it, with Navasana (The Boat Pose) ... the asana described next.

NAVASANA

The Boat Pose

NAVASANA (The Boat Pose) strengthens the lower back, while also toning and cleansing the muscles in the broad-expanse of the back and the legs. Additionally, Navasana enables one to fine-tune both a sense of balance and endurance.

1) Recline on the back, as in Savasana (the relaxation pose), but with the hands palms-down and the feet side-by-side and gently touching. Exhale slowly and consciously, and as you inhale …

2) Simultaneously lift the torso and the legs from the floor … each at about a 45^0 angle to the floor … and raise the arms so that they are straight and parallel to the floor. Try to keep the spine as straight as possible and not let it arch forward excessively. Keep the legs straight. Balance at a point between the lower back and the buttocks.

3) In the early stages of working with Navasana, retain the breath for 10 or 15 seconds and hold the posture. As strength, balance, and endurance increase, hold the posture for 30 or 40 seconds while breathing gently and abdominally. After holding the posture for an appropriate length of time, on a slow exhalation …

4) Release Navasana by slowly and simultaneously lowering the body, the legs, and the arms back to the floor.

5) Rest for a moment, after releasing the posture, by taking two or three slow, deep, complete inhalations. Then, on another inhalation …

6) Lift the body again to The Boat Pose, repeating the steps outlined above. Complete two to three rounds of the posture initially, eventually increasing to four or five rounds.

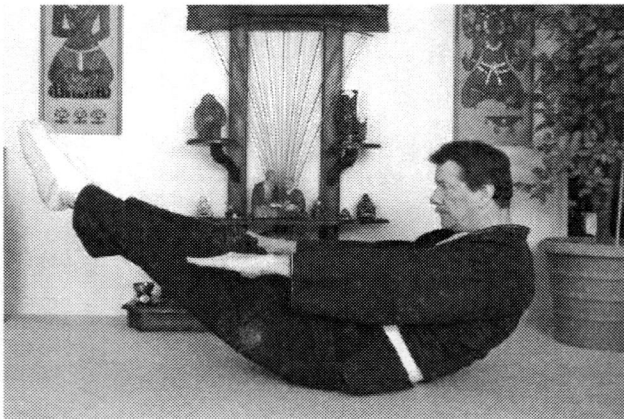

"When one is preoccupied not with Heaven, but is simply focused in the moment, then one is already *in* Heaven."

Helena Blavatsky

VIPARITA – KARANI

The Reverse Pose

The Reverse Pose flexes and strengthens the back, spine, and neck. With the body inverted, blood flows freely into the head, brain, and upper organs of the body. The thyroid gland in the throat, and the pituitary gland in the brain, especially benefit from this inverse relationship with gravity.

1) Recline on the back in Savasana (the relaxation posture). Exhale completely, releasing all tension. As you inhale ...

2) Lift first one, and then the other, leg off of the floor. Roll the hips off the floor (if possible), and bring the hands to the hips to help support the body.

3) Balance in the Reverse Pose with the feet just above, or slightly beyond, the head. Relax the breathing, focus the awareness on, and feel, the posture. Rest in the asana for 30 seconds to a minute, initially ... 1 to 3 minutes eventually.

4) Release the posture by either slowly lowering the straightened legs to the floor (if back strength permits), or bend the knees and fold the legs into the body and *roll* the spine back to the floor slowly ... lift the head from the floor (to prevent back strain), if necessary, as you roll the body down.

5) Always follow Viparita Karani with a back arch or two, or with Matsyasana (the Fish Posture). Rest for several minutes in Savasana.

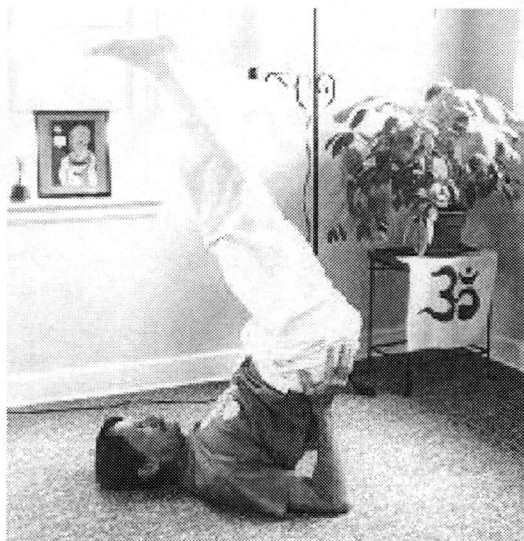

The Back Arch

&

MATSYASANA

The Fish Pose

Both Matsyasana (The Fish Pose) and The Back Arch facilitate deep, vigorous breathing by increasing flexibility in the neck, chest, and abdomen. Suppleness is also enhanced and maintained in the lower spine. Matsyasana is usually practiced following the inversion postures and prior to resting in Savasana.

Back Arch -

1) Lie on the back with legs together, knees bent, and the feet flat on the floor. Exhale completely. As you inhale ...

2) Arch back and buttocks off the floor as high as is comfortably possible.

3) Retain the breath and the posture for about 15 seconds. Exhale; lower the back to the floor, releasing the posture. Tense the abdominal muscles and press the small of the back into the floor. Hold for several seconds and release.

4) Repeat the back arch two or three times ... perhaps holding the asana the final time for about 30 seconds with relaxed breathing.

Matsyasana -

1) Lie on the back with the legs folded/crossed ... as if sitting in a cross-legged posture. Place the hands under the thighs, palms up, so the arms can be used for support. Exhale completely. As you inhale ...

2) Arch the spine and drop the head back so that the body rests on the buttocks and the top of the head, supported by forearms and elbows.

3) Breathe deeply and completely ... focus the awareness on the throat. Visualize as if breathing directly into and out of the throat ... as if the throat has nostrils. Hold the asana for about 5 to 7 deep, complete breaths. Release on an exhalation.

4) Place the hands at the back of the head and lift the head, bringing the chin to the chest. Hold for several seconds, vigorously stretching the muscles of the neck. Release. Rest the head on the floor, straighten the legs, and rest in Savasana for several minutes.

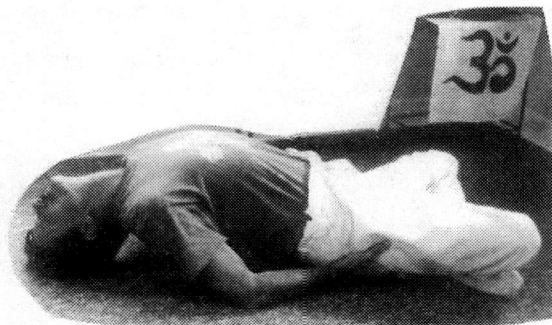

Intermediate Postures

Most of the postures and techniques of the yogas are really quite simple... *deceptively* simple, in a way ... hard to believe that such simplicity can so profoundly affect mind and body. Yet, the proof is in the practice. In a relatively short period of time, one can positively and personally *experience* the results of a regular practice. However, if one tends more toward the scientific, there are many books readily available that examine yoga in a clinical light.

After practicing the postures described in the first part of this book for awhile, the student might find greater challenges to their liking. These postures should be practiced, as with all of Hatha Yoga, gently and with discretion. No one practice is right for everyone. As with all of the physical techniques of Hatha Yoga, they should be practiced slowly and conscientiously, with full awareness of movements into the posture, with awareness of the maintenance of the posture, and awareness of the movements releasing the posture. Slow, conscientious, and deliberate movements are important! The movements should be graceful ... *grace*-**filled**! A practice should never be rushed. The practice of the yogas is outside of linear time. Even though our schedule may only allow a few postures at a time, after awhile we begin to experience the "yoga" in everything we do throughout the course of the day ... driving the car ... washing dishes ... working in the yard ... human interaction ... in ways far beyond Hatha Yoga.

Slow, conscientious, deliberate movements gives the mind the time necessary to fully enter into the experience of the moment. Remember: yoga is always practiced as a *meditation*! We are not mindlessly assuming a posture as thoughts wander elsewhere. Rather, the mind must be *in* the posture! ... and what that means is that we use the sense-sations as focal points for the mind. We *feel* the stretching muscles and the gently realigning skeletal system of the body. With the power of visualization, we *see* the body in its posture ... as if we were standing a few feet from it and looking back at it ... as if the body were at the center of a sphere, with the vision on the surface of the sphere, rotating around the body, seeing it from all angles ... from all sides.

On a practical level, slow movements enable one to stop or limit a posture if the body is sending a caution signal. If one moves rapidly into a posture, and overdoes it, the harm is already done before there is time to modify. Thus: s-l-o-w and conscious ...

The beauties of the yogas are that they are spiritual, they are mindful, they are practical. They apply to, and work with, every level of existence ... from the esoteric to the mundane. The question, then, isn't whether or not we practice yoga, but rather whether or not we know what yoga we're practicing!

N A T A R A J A S A N A

The Dancing Shiva

Natarajasana helps develop balance and poise. As one rests and stretches comfortably in the Dancing Shiva, the mind becomes still and serene. Leg muscles are fortified, the rib cage is expanded, and the vertebral joints and muscles surrounding the spine are stretched and strengthened.

1) Assume a standing posture and lean slightly to the left (you can begin on either side), shifting the body's weight to align over that leg.

2) Lean slightly forward as you bend the right knee and rest the right foot in the right hand. Pull up on the right foot, using the principle of isometrics - pushing against the hand with the foot and pulling against the foot with the hand.

3) Extend the left arm at a slight upward angle (about 45 degrees), straighten the fingers, and bend the wrist back vigorously.

4) Balance in the posture for 45 seconds to a minute. Let the breath be gentle and abdominal.

5) Release Natarajasana on an exhalation. Repeat the asana reversing the arm and leg positions.

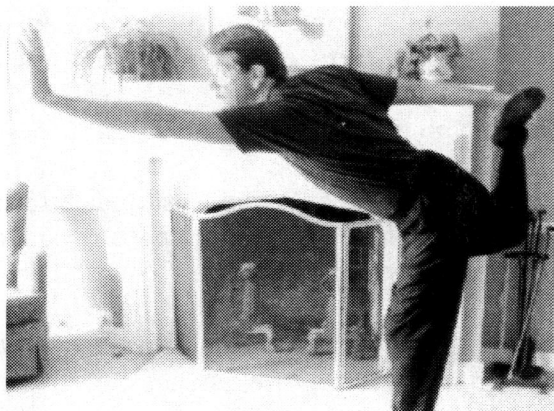

"My soul is my counsel and has taught me to give ear to the voices which are created neither by tongues nor uttered by throats. Now I can listen to silence with serenity and can hear in that silence the hymns of ages chanting exaltations to the sky and revealing the secrets of eternity."

Kahlil Gibran

VERIBHADRASANA

The Hero Pose

Veribhadrasana complements, and is often practiced following, the Triangle pose (Trikonasana). The Hero pose is a balancing posture that greatly strengthens the legs (mainly the thighs), the lower back, and the neck, and increases flexibility in the arms and shoulders.

1) Stand straight with the feet about a yard apart and the arms hanging relaxed at the sides. Exhale completely. On a deep, complete inhalation ...

2) Lift and vigorously stretch the arms straight overhead, palms together, fingers pointing toward the ceiling.

3) Turn the body, and the left foot, 90° to the left. As you exhale ...

4) Bend the left knee until the left leg forms a right angle, with the left thigh parallel to the floor. Keep the right leg straight (if possible) as it slides back, and keep the right knee off the floor, adjust the right foot to complement the balance. The head remains erect, and the arms remain stretched overhead, fingers pointing toward the ceiling.

Hold the posture for 5 to 10 seconds, initially ... 20 to 30 seconds eventually. Exhale completely, and on an inhalation ...

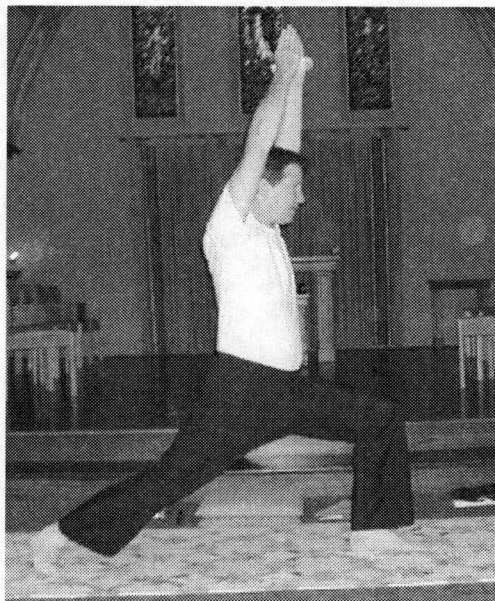

5) Straighten the left leg slowly and lift the body. Turn to the right; as you exhale …

6) Repeat the posture on the opposite side.

Advanced Postures

Having developed a degree of
proficiency with the postures of
earlier sections of this book,
you may want to ease into working with
some of the more advanced poses.

However, the advanced postures should
be considered simply an *option*.

Certain limitations of the body
may not make working with advanced
postures practical at this time.

What is important is knowing that continuous
work with the basic postures, presented
earlier in this book, is perfectly sufficient
for creating the environment necessary
to health, awareness, and realization.

SARVANGASANA

The Shoulder Stand

Sarvangasana is purported to positively affect virtually the entire physiological system. The Sanskrit word "sarvang" literally means "all parts". The effect on the skeletal system is readily apparent: the spine, especially at the neck, is greatly strengthened, and full flexibility is retained. Inverting the body also profoundly affects circulation; cleansing, nourishing, and refreshing blood flows effortlessly into the upper organs on the body ... assisted now, rather than hindered, by the force of gravity. Additionally, Sarvangasana, when coupled with Matsyasana (The Fish Pose) is said to rejuvenate and stimulate the Thyroid gland ... a very essential part of the body's regulatory system. When the endocrine (glandular) system is functioning properly and harmoniously, one's moods are calmed and balanced ... and when the moods are calmed and balanced, the work with the mind naturally deepens and intensifies.

1) Recline on the back in Savasana (the Relaxation Posture). Exhale. On an inhalation lift first one, then the other, leg off the floor, assuming Viparita Karani (the Reverse Pose).

2) Hold the Reverse Pose for approximately 30 seconds, then, on an exhalation, bend and lower the knees to the forehead. Body weight is now shifted primarily to the shoulders and neck, and the chin is near, or touching, the chest.

3) On an inhalation, slowly extend and straighten the legs, keeping the back as straight as possible. Relax the breathing and hold the posture ... initially for 30 seconds to a minute; eventually, 3 to 5 minutes.

VARIATION: If the legs are very vertical and the body feels comfortably balanced, try extending the arms adjacent to the sides, balancing entirely on the shoulders, the neck, and the back of the head.

4) After the posture has been maintained for an appropriate period of time, lower one leg overhead, on an exhalation, bringing the toes as close to the floor as possible. Inhale and lift the leg back to its vertical position. Repeat with the other leg. Then, on an exhalation, lower both feet overhead to Halasana (the Plow Pose ... see next asana).

5) If both feet are on the floor in Halasana, stretch vigorously ... with legs straight, push the feet as far from the head as possible. The flex and stretch in the back and neck may be even further increased by bending and lowering the knees to the floor.

6) On an exhalation lower the hips, lifting the feet from the floor and, in a continuous motion, inhale extending the body once again to Sarvangasana. Hold for another 30 seconds to a minute.

7) Release the posture on an exhalation. To further increase spinal flexibility, place the hands at the lower back thus creating a vigorous arch (Setu Bandhasana - the Bridge Pose) as the feet are returned to the starting position. Hold the Bridge Pose for several seconds, then release on an exhalation.

8) Always follow Sarvangasana with Matsyasana (the Fish Pose) in order to fully balance the effectiveness of the work on the thyroid gland and the throat. Matsyasana should be held for the time it takes to complete five to ten deep, slow breaths ... with awareness focused in the throat. Visualize as if the throat has nostrils and you are breathing directly into and out of the throat ... this visualization effectively focuses the energies in the throat.

9) After the Fish Pose is released, fold the legs over the chest, wrap the arms around the shins, and lift the head to the knees ... gently flexing the body in the Cradle Pose for about 30 seconds.

10) On an exhalation, release the Cradle Pose and fully extend the body to Savasana (the Relaxation Posture).

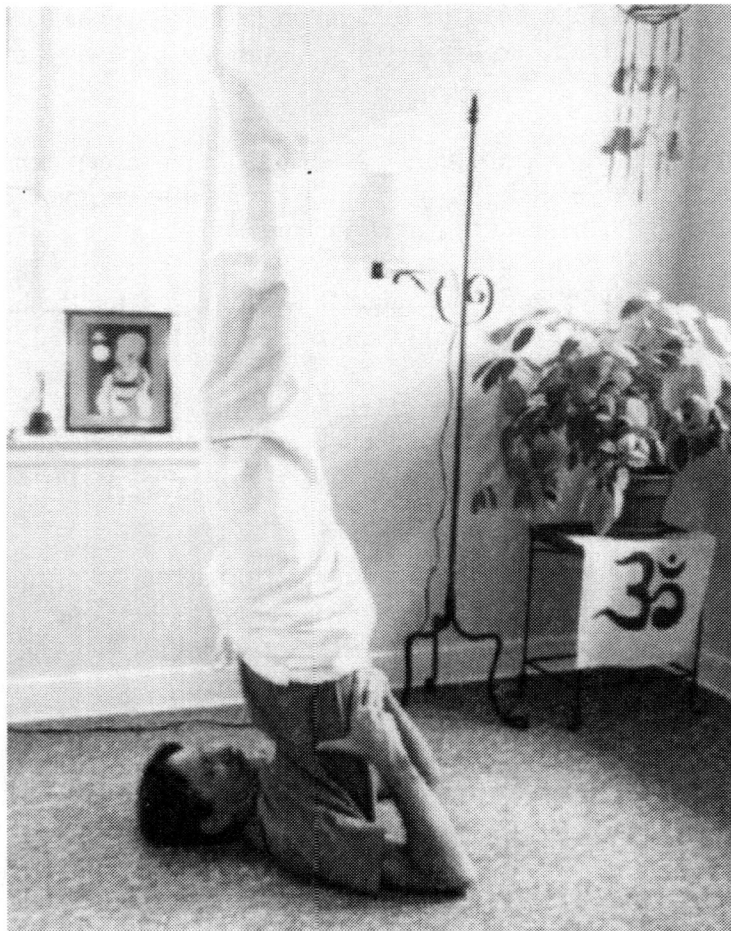

Sarvangasana

HALASANA

The Plow Pose

Many of the benefits of Pashimatana (the Head- to-Knee posture) and the inversion postures are offered in Halasana. Most profoundly, the Plow Pose creates and maintains flexibility in the neck, and stimulates and affects harmonious functioning in the thyroid and parathyroid glands of the throat.

Halasana may be practiced as an independent posture; however, it usually complements Sarvangasana (the Shoulder Stand).

1) Recline on the back, assuming the Relaxation posture, Savasana. Exhale completely. As you inhale ...

2) Lift first one, and then the other, leg from the floor, rolling the hips off the floor ... as if assuming Viparita Karani (the Reverse pose), but continue the overhead movement, bringing the feet to, or as close to, the floor as is comfortably possible. Keep the legs as straight as possible.

Note: the feet may not, and need not, come all the way to the floor ... but keep the legs straight.

3) Rest in Halasana for thirty seconds to a minute, initially ... a minute to three minutes, eventually ... with the breathing relaxed and diaphragmatic.

4) Release the posture on an exhalation. Methods of release vary, depending on the strength of the lower back ... take precautions to avoid strain in the lower back. The least strenuous method for the release of Halasana (and Sarvangasana ... the Shoulder Stand) is to fold the legs into the chest and roll the body back to the floor, lifting the head from the floor. The most back-strengthening method is to release the posture by lowering the straightened legs slowly back to the floor.

To effect proper balance in the work with the thyroid glands, always follow Halasana with Matsyasana (the Fish pose).

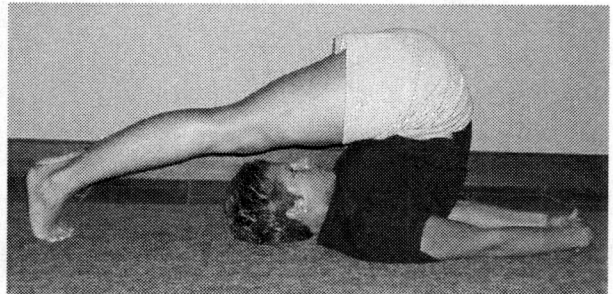

"That which is simple is simply seen.
But know that there are those who so mask themselves,
That, for them, what is simple is rarely understood."

Master Po

USTRASANA

The Camel

The Camel Pose vigorously arches the spine, and stimulates circulation in the spinal cord and nerve ganglia. It stretches the chest muscles, and develops and maintains suppleness, strength, and flexibility in the knees. Circulation is stimulated in the throat and head.

1) Begin in a kneeling pose ... with the torso and thighs upright and vertical. The knees and ankles should be touching, or very slightly apart. Take a deep, complete inhalation, and then ...

2) As you exhale, lean back, arch the spine, and bring the hands to rest on the heels, or ankles if possible. (Note: suppleness and flexibility vary greatly; initially it may be necessary to support the body by placing the hands on the hips or on the backs of the thighs.)

3) Let the head drop back freely. Gently clench the teeth together, so that the throat is stretched vigorously.

4) With the breathing calm and relaxed, rest in the posture for 15 to 30 seconds, initially ... increasing to 40 seconds to a minute, eventually. Alternately focus the awareness in the spine and in the throat.

5) Release the Camel Pose on an inhalation ... pulling the body back upright, from the base of the spine. In a continuous motion, and on an exhalation, fold the body to the Fallen Leaf posture (Balasana). Rest and relax for about a minute before continuing with your practice.

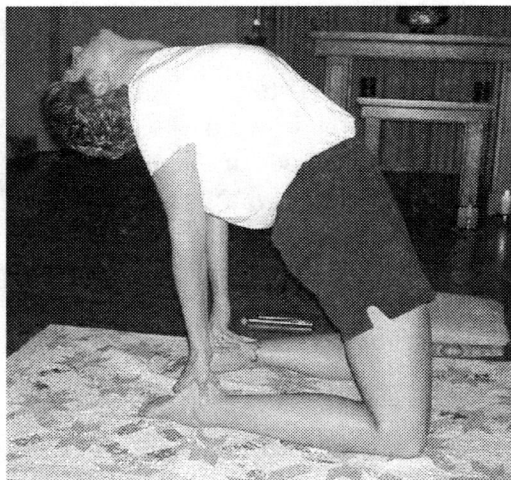

"I like boring things. I like things to be exactly the same over and over again because the more you look at the same thing, the more the meaning goes away, and the better and emptier you feel."

Andy Warhol

SIRSHASANA

The Headstand

Sirshasana (The Headstand) is perhaps the posture most associated with yoga. This powerful asana stimulates a fresh and free-flowing supply of blood to the upper organs: the thyroid gland (in the throat), the eyes, ears, and, perhaps most significantly, the brain. The skeletal system of the neck is greatly strengthened, as are the muscles in the neck, back, arms, and shoulders. Sirshasana is also a superb posture in which to discover and develop the control and balance essential to life.

This version of Headstand is executed in four stages. These stages may be practiced as individual asanas (postures); or they may be executed in a series of flowing movements resulting in the full headstand.

First-quarter Headstand -

1) Begin sitting in Vajrasana (see page 3).

2) Lift the body up on the knees and bend forward from the waist; place the elbows and forearms on the floor. To assure proper positioning, the hands should just reach the opposite elbow if the forearms are turned inward.

3) With the elbows in proper position, bring the hands together, intertwine the fingers, and form an open "cup" with the hands.

4) Place the head on the floor, about midway between the crown and the forehead, so that it rests in the cup formed by the hands.

5) Straighten the knees and lift the body, forming an inverted "V"; press the heels toward the floor. Hold 30 seconds to one minute.

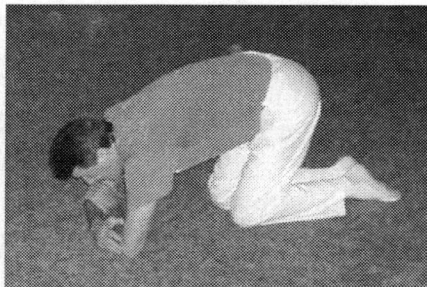

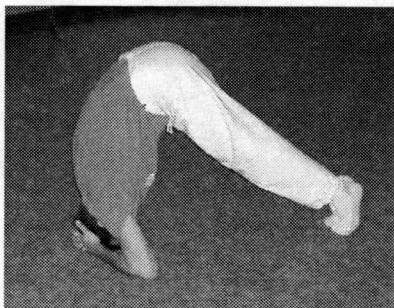

This is the First-quarter Headstand posture. Flow of blood to the head is stimulated and the hamstring muscles are stretched.

To increase strength in the arms and shoulders, while in this posture:

55

5a) Lift the head from the floor and look down at the hands for several seconds, then lower the head back to the hands. Rest, then repeat four or five times.

5b) Bring the knees back to the floor and rest for about a minute in the Fallen Leaf Posture.

5c) Curl the body s-l-o-w-l-y to Vajrasana.

Important: It may be necessary to work with the First-quarter Headstand for days ... or even weeks ... to develop the upper-body strength needed for the following stages of Headstand. Even if one never works beyond the First-quarter Posture, just this degree of Headstand is an effective and powerful asana which one should continue to practice!

Second-quarter Headstand -

Bring the body to position 5) described in First-quarter Headstand:

5) Straighten the knees and lift the body, forming the inverted "V" mentioned above; press the heels toward the floor.

6) "Walk" toward the head, increasing the sharpness of the "V", and increasing the degree of stretch in the hamstring muscles and the vertical pitch of the back.

7) Gently lift the feet off the floor, fold the legs toward the chest and balance on the head and forearms.

This is the Second-quarter Headstand. The body is inverted, the legs are bent at the knees, and the thighs are tucked in towards the chest. Work with this posture until you can hold and balance in it for thirty seconds to one full minute.

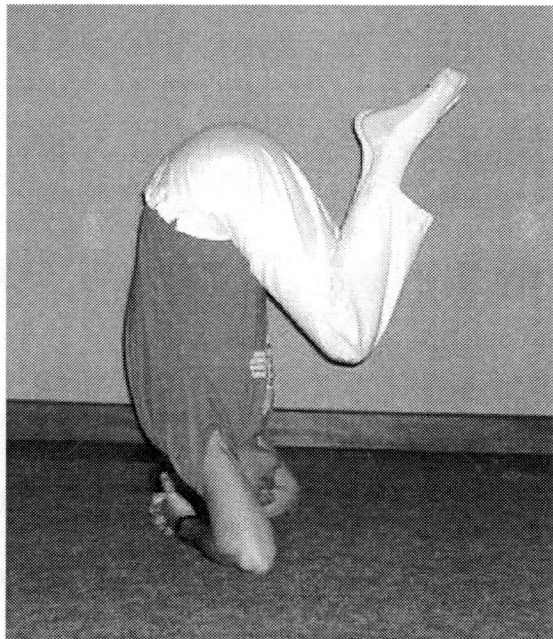

Third-quarter Headstand -

8) Straighten the legs at the hips so that the head, torso, and thighs form a vertical line. The legs are still bent at the knees.

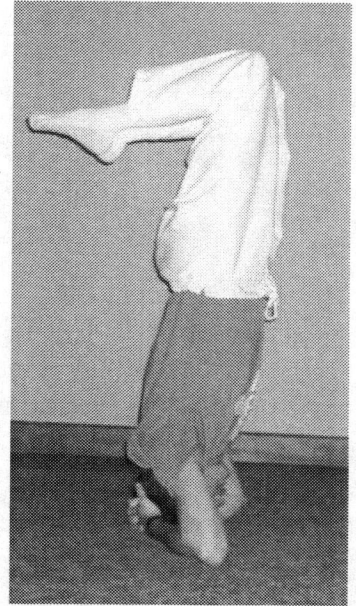

Full Headstand -

9) Gently, slowly, and fully straighten the legs.

Much of the essence of Headstand is the development of strength and execution of *controlled movements*. Therefore, each of the first three quarters of this asana should be held for at least 10 seconds before moving on to the subsequent postures.

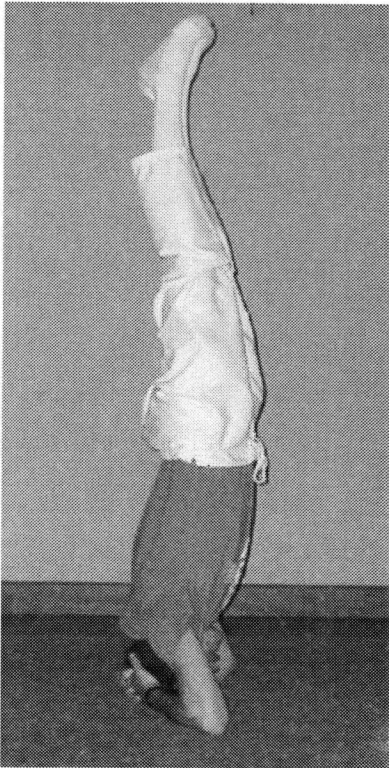

Exiting Headstand -

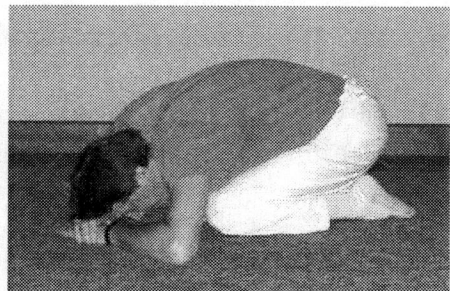

10) To release the Headstand, reverse the movements of the preceding stages ... slowly and with control ... holding each quarter posture for 5 to 10 seconds.

11) Once the body returns to the floor, rest in the Fallen Leaf pose for about a minute before s-l-o-w-l-y curling the body to Vajrasana sitting posture.

KAKASANA

The Crow Pose

Kakasana (The Crow Pose) develops strength in the arms and wrists and creates powerful stomach and abdominal muscles. The posture also assists in developing the balance essential to the execution of Sirshasana (The Headstand) and to the overall establishment of a calm center of mind.

1) Sit in a squatting position; feet as flat on the floor as possible.

2) Lean forward and position the arms between the knees. Place the palms of the hands flat on the floor with the fingers turned slightly in, elbows slightly bent, and rest the knees firmly just above the elbows.

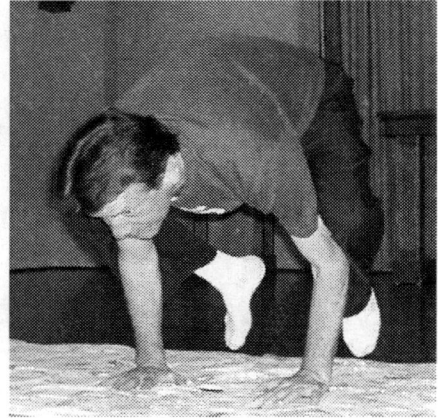

3) Slowly, with strength and control, lean forward lifting the feet off the floor until the body is supported by the hands and forearms. Hold the posture as long as possible ... to a maximum of 30 seconds ... with gentle, abdominal breathing.

VARIATION:

4) Assume the starting posture described in #1 above, but ...

5) Place both legs to the left side of the left arm, resting the right knee just above the left elbow.

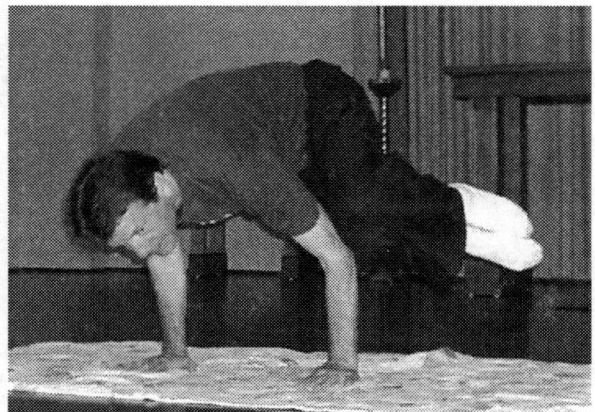

6) Lean slowly to the right and lift both legs and feet off of the floor. Hold the posture as long as possible ... a maximum of 30 seconds ... with gentle abdominal breathing.

7) Repeat the posture on the right side.

HANSASANA

The Swan

&

MAYURASANA

The Peacock

Hanurasana (The Swan) is a balancing and strengthening posture.

Mayurasana (The Peacock) complements and enhances the dynamics of The Swan.

Both postures tone and strengthen the abdominal organs by applying vigorous intra-abdominal pressure. The liver, pancreas, stomach, and kidneys directly benefit, and circulation to the head is greatly stimulated. When the posture and pressure are released, fresh blood rushes to, and flushes, the organs of the digestive system.

HANSASANA (The Swan) -

1) Assume a kneeling position and separate the knees to about shoulder width. Place the hands flat on the floor with fingers pointing back.

2) Bring the elbows as close together as is comfortably possible, and lower the abdomen to the elbows.

3) Lean forward and bring the forehead to the floor, straighten the legs, and curl the toes under.

4) On an inhalation, arch the head up and back (as in Cobra). Relax the breathing and hold the posture for several seconds.

5) Release the asana on an exhalation. Fold the body to rest in the Fallen Leaf pose.

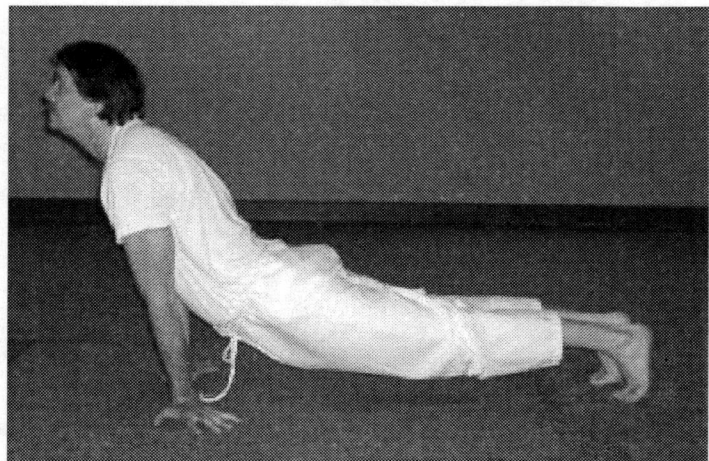

MAYURASANA (The Peacock) - Repeat steps 1 through 3 of The Swan.

1) Instead of fully arching the head and neck, simply raise the head until it is parallel to the floor.

2) Shift the body's weight forward and lift the feet off the floor, balancing entirely on the forearms and elbows.

3) Arch the spine vigorously, lifting the feet as high as is comfortably possible. Allow the forehead to rest lightly on the floor.

4) Hold for several seconds, then release the asana on an exhalation. Fold the body to rest in Balasana ... the Fallen Leaf posture.

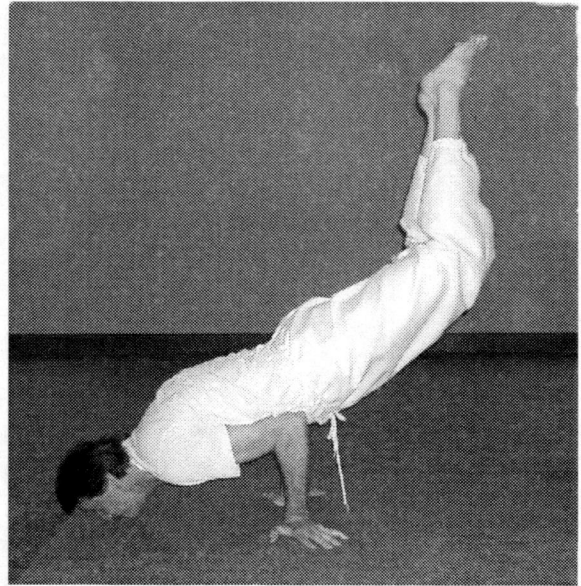

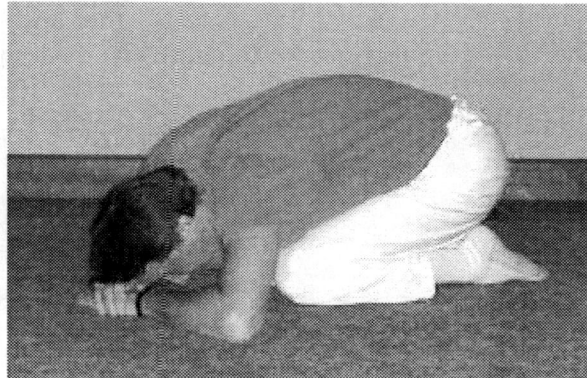

"There is no failure as long as we continue to make an effort."

Patanjali

SUPTA – VAJRASANA

The Kneeling Stretch

Supta-Vajrasana (The Kneeling Stretch) is an abdomen-stimulating exercise. This posture encourages vigorous circulation in the principle nerve center of the body: the solar plexus (Manipura Chakra). The adrenal glands are stimulated, and the thigh muscles are firmed and toned. Flexibility in the knee joints is maintained, and the rib-cage is expanded.

1) Sit on the floor in the Diamond Pose (Vajrasana). Separate the knees and feet so that the buttocks rests on the floor. (If you cannot sit comfortably in this variation, then simply sit in Vajrasana.) Hold this posture for 30 seconds to one minute.

2) As the stretch in the leg muscles increases, and the body begins to rest comfortably, lean back, supporting the body on the elbows, and thus increasing the thigh stretch and knee flex.

3) Continue to recline ... to the floor, if possible, holding full Supta-Vajrasana for 30 seconds to one minute.

4) After releasing the posture, sit with the legs straight for several seconds to relieve the stretching tension in the muscles and to allow normal circulation to return to the legs.

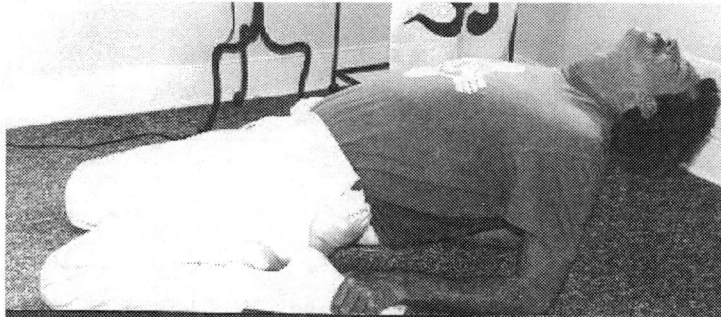

"But if the things of my dreams are real, where are they now?" Carlos asked his teacher, Juan Matus.

"They are here," don Juan replied. "And if you had the power, you could call them back. But now you cannot do that because you think it is helpful to maintain a doubting, nagging, questioning mind. It isn't, my friend ... it isn't. There are worlds upon worlds right here in front of us. You will reap their benefit when you learn to relax in, and accept, this world."

From "A Yaqui Way of Knowledge" by Carlos Casteneda

Suggested Hatha Yoga Routine

1) **SITTING & CENTERING:** Begin sitting in the comfortable posture of your choice ... cross-legged or The Diamond Pose (Vajrasana). Let the breathing become relaxed and abdominal. Focus the awareness on the scalp, and slowly move the awareness down...through the face, torso, arms and hands, and into the legs and feet – *visualize* the relaxed muscles as you proceed. (If you wish, complement visualization with neck and/or breathing exercises.)

2) **SITTING TWISTS & STRETCHING ROUTINE:**

    A) Pashimatana (Head-to-knee posture)
    B) Bhodi-konasana (Butterfly pose)
    C) Janu-sirasana (Head-to-knee w/one leg straight)
    D) Ardha-matsyendrasana (Half twist)

3) **STOMACH-RECLINING & KNEELING EXERCISES:**

    A) Salabasanas (Locust poses)
    B) Bhujangasana (Cobra pose)
    C) Supta-Vajrasana (Diamond pose variation)
    D) Ustrasana (Camel pose)
    E) Fallen Leaf ... then, slow-curl to Vajrasana

4) **STANDING ROUTINE:** Stand & Center in a firm, but restful and relaxed, posture following the routine suggested in SITTING & CENTERING above. Then ...

    A) Padahastasana (Standing head-to-knee)
    B) Trikonasana (Triangle pose)
    C) Veribhadrasana (Hero pose)
    D) Surya Namaskar (The Sun Salutation)

5) **BACK-RECLINING EXERCISES:**

    A) Viparita Karani/Sarvangasana (Reverse/Shoulderstand postures)
    B) Halasana (Plow pose) ... then return to inversion posture
    C) Matsyasana (Fish pose)
    D) Reclining Simple Twist (knees bent, feet on floor, arms extended; legs & head fall/twist in opposite direction) & Cradle posture. Conclude with ...

6) **SAVASANA** (Deep relaxation): Recline on the back with arms extended adjacent to the sides, let the breath be calm and abdominal. Practice resting *consciously* ... **not** falling asleep ... canvass the body with awareness - use the power of visualization to "*see*", as well as feel, the body at rest. After canvassing the body with awareness, simply focus the awareness on the gentle rising and falling of the abdomen. And rest.

Part II

The Mind of Yoga

The Philosophies of Yoga

To consider Hatha Yoga to be all of yoga
would be to consider P.E. to be all of school.

Hatha yoga is the physical system
that enables one to more fully
practice the yogas of mind … and beyond.

This enables us to
discover the philosophies of yoga …
which ultimately lead to a deeper understanding
of *how* the universe is …
and *why* it is as it is …
and our role in it.

Choice

As fascinating as it is to watch a bird build its nest, in fact, it cannot do otherwise. As beautiful as is the bee's hive, it cannot choose to do differently. The spider has no alternative but to weave its web.

But we have **choice** ... *conscious* choice. We can choose to walk into a river and try in vain to push it back upstream, if we want to. Or we can choose to walk into the river, lift our feet from the river floor, and float effortlessly downstream. We can choose to be conscious of obstacles in our path and navigate around them; or we can choose to be *un*-conscious ... and collide with everything. In fact, we can choose not to enter the river at all! We can just sit safely and idly on its bank and watch it flow for awhile. We can *stay* on the bank, if we so chose, and miss the journey completely ... with all of its suffering ... *and* with all of its pleasures.

We can choose to feel the Summer sun's warmth or the cool Autumn rain on our skin, and we can choose to *marvel* at that sensation. Or we can choose to believe the words of others when they tell us how miserable the weather is.

With the same freedom of Spirit with which we can choose destruction, we can also choose creation. The choice is ours. The choice is *always* ours.

Our choices determine who we are. ***And who we are is our gift to others.***

Being At Peace

If you wish to live in a world of peace, then *be* at peace. Sound simple? *Is* it that simple?

"Peace on earth …" is a phrase we hear often during The Holiday Season. Almost everyone agrees on the desirability of peace on earth. It's given a lot of Christmas-time lip service. However, *arriving* at The Place of Peace is another matter. Arriving at that place as an individual is tough enough, but how can we get the whole *world* to be at peace? What a monumental task! How do we achieve **Peace On Earth**?

The "how" part of "peace on earth" is really quite simple, as it turns out. Of course, what is *simple* and what is *easy* are not always one and the same.

Ram Dass and others have observed: "The only work we have to do is on our self." First, we must come to understand that statement. We have to redirect our focus from "out there" to "in here". If we want peace on earth, we must *be* at peace. Here is one technique for realizing that objective. It is a simple, yet effective, ages-old technique:

Sit comfortably, either on the floor or in a chair, so that the head, neck, and spine are in alignment. Do what you can to create a restful environment. Accept the presence of whatever is *in* the moment, yet *out* of your direct, personal control … such as the usual sounds of passing cars and chirping birds and people in the distance laughing and talking. Bring the awareness into the moment by slowly moving from sense to sense. The mind usually wants to focus on all of the problems it thinks it has, but by focusing the awareness on the sense-sations of the moment, the mind is gently prevented from becoming stressed. *Feel* the body in its sitting posture … as if the body were sitting for the first time. Feel the points of contact with the floor or the chair; feel the force of gravity on the body … creating the *illusion* of weight. Begin to gradually see through the illusions … including, and especially, the illusion that peace isn't already here! Just notice the light falling on the eyelids. Do not desire that the moment be other than it is; rather, just discover it just *as* it is. Be passively aware of the sounds falling on the ears. Notice the smells; taste the tastes. Pretend you're a visitor from another planet who has just inhabited a body for the first time and you don't even know what to *expect*. Pretend that you don't even know what experience is desirable or undesirable. *Feel* the breath flowing gently into and out of the body … *feel* the abdomen slowly expanding and relaxing with each gentle, calm breath.

Take a moment to *discover* the moment! Rather than trying to define it, manipulate it, or judge it, as we so often do, just passively notice it. Begin to discover the perfection in even the moments that are not of your personal liking.

Yoga and meditation mean being <u>in</u> the moment … just as it is … not trying to make it the way we want it to be, but discovering it as it is, and even *accepting* it as it is. This doesn't mean that we don't sometimes work for change; it means that there are *ways* to change what is without creating resistance or attachments. We begin to learn how to get *un*constructive things out of our life without pushing, and we begin to learn how to get *con*structive things into our life without creating clinging.

As we sit and practice the simple exercise described above, it may be that our body is surrounded by noise and turmoil. A construction crew may be working nearby; there may be traffic noise; we may be sitting directly beneath an airport landing zone. It may be too hot, or too cold. But if we are just being *with* the moment, then how could we possibly be "distracted"? Distracted from *what*? From The Moment? Whatever we think would distract us is the moment! If we're just being with what *is*, and if what is, is what we are gently focused on, then peace is all that's possible!

By the same token, we may be in the most idyllic of settings - warm Spring day, with the sun and the breeze alternately warming and cooling the skin, and hearing only the sounds of birds' songs and, perhaps, a babbling brook nearby, or the leaves rustling in the wind - but if there is inner turmoil, then there is no peace.

Our most common error is in thinking we must *create* peace. We give ourselves an impossible task, and then lament that it's *impossible*! We need only *be* at peace. We're enabling the peace that *is* – to *be*! It's so simple! But individual and collective psychology makes it, at the same time, so very difficult to realize.

Our environment, and our surroundings may *complement* our peace ... but they cannot create it ... nor can they destroy it. The Kingdom is within. The choice is ours. The choice is *always* ours.

If you want Peace On Earth, you must first: Be At Peace!

Creating an Environment

What we are doing in a yoga practice is creating an environment in which the truth ... the truth that we *are* ... can flow through us. Just that. We are not *doing* something in a traditional sense ... in the sense that we are accustomed to "doing". It is not *accomplishment* in the sense of building a bridge or completing a project. And that is what is so hard for most minds to comprehend. That is why it is so important to create and establish a practice ... and to keep working with that practice. Keep working with it, regardless of how one "feels" about it at the moment ... regardless of whether or not one is "in the mood" or "wants to". That is why it is so important to *not* look for results ... but rather, to simply create a setting ... an environment ... in which results can *reveal* themselves. To the extent we are attached to concepts such as "progress" and "improvement" and "achievement" ... and all of the mind-set that accompanies these concepts ... we will be eternally disappointed, and the practice will certainly cease, because the results will never be quantitative enough ... they will never be timely enough ... never come fast enough ... be enough. Rather, we establish a practice and *just do it* (as the popular commercial advises) ... and allow the results to reveal themselves. Make no mistake about it: there *are* results! And they *will* be revealed! ... in time, and with practice. However, they are often not what we expected at all ... probably not what we were expecting! But they are *real* ... in time, and with practice.

Often, in class, I suggest, as we sit or stand with eyes closed, that we simply, passively gaze into the void ... *look* for nothing. Just look, passively, and see what is there. Like walking through a forest and simply noticing this tree or that tree ... this rock or that rock ... the sound of gravel crunching underfoot ... the smell of the air ... the feel of the sun, or the cool air, or both, on the skin. In a natural environment, like a forest or a beach, we're usually not busy *judging* what we see. We're not busy thinking, "If only that oak were a pine ... how much better it would be!" or "That maple would be much more attractive if only its branches were shaped like this or like that." Such judgments would be absurd, of course, and usually we know it. Instead, we tend to simply see the things of nature as they are ... accept nature as it is. It's not a matter of liking it or disliking it ... it's just **as it is**! And the practice we create and work with no matter what!, enables us to begin to rest in such a place, even while dealing with those things we do tend to judge ... such as other people ... such as our self ... such as circumstances.

We are like a musical instrument, in a way. After we listen to a beautiful piano piece, we don't walk up to the piano and compliment it! We may admire it as an instrument, and treat it with care and respect and appreciation for what it is. But regardless of how fine an instrument it is, we realize that the music simply *comes through it* ... that the music wasn't created *by* it. Likewise, as our practice deepens, and our environment becomes established, we begin to recognize and realize our worldly, material form – our body and our mind – as mere *instruments* through which our work, our purpose, and our offerings, flow. Our ego is still fully functional and intact, but becomes less relevant.

The yoga and meditation Master, Suzuki Roshi, once wrote a book called "Beginners Mind". In this book he suggests one learn to always maintain the mind of the "beginner". Never seek to become an expert, he advises. In our culture, of course, that probably sounds like absurd advice! Everything many of us are about in this worldly setting is *perfecting* our self ... becoming an expert. And, at the worldly level, that is indeed what the game is all about. But when seen through the eyes of a yoga practitioner, Suzuki's words are exquisitely wise.

Imagine two individuals walking into a forest: one is an expert biologist, in search of a specific specimen; the other is someone walking into a forest for the very first time ... perhaps a young child. The "expert" rejects this and this and this ... pushes aside what does not fit the criterion of what is being sought. But the newcomer to the forest, the child's mind, rejects nothing! The newcomer isn't "looking for" anything. The new-comer is just *discovering*. Looking for nothing ... open to discovering *everything*! There isn't anything that doesn't fit the "criterion" of the beginner, because there is no criterion! It's all taken in. It all fits ... equally. As in meditation we gaze into the void: looking for nothing ... finding everything.

At a worldly level, it is wonderful that a researcher, like a biologist, looks discriminately ... and rejects this and this and this. Because we want the researcher to find specifically what he or she is looking for so that they can apply it to science and fulfill the objective of "researching". Although this is not the goal of a yoga practice, it is often our mind-set. We are not trying to *improve* our lot (although that may have been our initial motivation for beginning a practice in the first place), we are simply *discovering* our lot ... passively ... and allowing that passive discovery to reveal Ultimate Purpose.

"Hold lightly to *beliefs*!", I advise yoga students. "Attachments to belief systems can im-prison us. Focus, rather, on what you *discover*!" Suppose you don't believe in gravity ... but then you walk off of a tall building. What happens next is not at all dependent on what you believe! I frequently hear people say, "I don't believe in this or that." And I say, "What does what you believe in have to do with anything?" It's fine to have beliefs. There are things I believe ... but at the same time I recognize that "belief" is simply the mind's way of attempting to make sense of it all. It's just the mind's way of saying, "This is how I *think* it is." That's fine. It's comforting to the mind to begin to believe it has the mysteries all figured out. That is what the mind thinks the purpose of the world is in the first place: something to be figured out. But the yogi remains always open to the possibility that he or she just very well may be totally and completely *wrong*! If one is not attached to beliefs and discovers he is wrong, there is no problem ... he simply keeps working, but with new data. If one *is* attached to beliefs and discovers he is wrong, then the suffering is great (or the denial is great) and the work probably comes to a screeching halt. The discovery is given a label, like "evil" or "demonic" ... or some label that justifies to the mind discontinuing the practice ... the search ... and returning to what Ram Dass calls "the practical neuroses of life".

Maybe, when I die, I will go to a big, golden gate and be admitted to (or not) Heaven. Maybe I will cycle around again and come back to this plane over and over and over again. Maybe I'll be sent straight to Hell. I don't know. It is as it is. I may *think* or *believe* it is this way or that way ... but it is as it is. Why should I even think I *have* to know? Rather, as a yogi, I seek only ... and *simply* ... to do the work that lies before me. And whatever lies before me *is* the work! And what I discover is what I discover. I seek only to create the environment. That is all that is required of me. The truth and the answers will be revealed when I am ready to hear them ... to see them ... to know them ... when I am capable of recognizing them. They're already right in front of me ... and you! They're already *here* ... *now*. I ready myself to receive them by doing the work ... by creating the environment. It is a deliciously "vicious" cycle!

The TAO

In Eastern philosophy, a concept of "reality" is called The Tao (pronounced: dow).

Tao is life experienced as flowing movement ... as neutral power, like wind or water. "The Tao" translates: "The Way", and one who is in accord with it is said to be in a perpetual state of grace.

Experiencing this perpetual grace means knowing relaxation-in-action ... freedom from craving ... understanding that we *are* it all already ... that it is only our *belief* in limitation that separates us from harmony ... and conquering that negative belief. Our belief in separateness manifests itself as ego-assertiveness ... as aggression... and as a desire to possess life in fixed forms of concepts and ideas. Thus, the ancient axiom: "Attachments to beliefs will imprison you. Let the attachments go. Free yourself that you may *dis*-cover - *un*-cover - truth."

One method for realizing non-assertiveness and non-aggression is the practice of meditation ... in which we learn to relax in *all* settings. As breathing is systematically relaxed and the mind gently focused on the calm breath, our grasp on desires is naturally released ... we let go. We become passive, but with firm resolve ... passive in *expectations* ... not necessarily passive in actions.

When one is relaxed with the natural elements ... flowing with the wind and water and the nature of humankind, one is at peace with The Way It Is ... with whatever life offers. Then ego-assertiveness and aggression are easily released. We become as a pillar of granite ... negativity, with no place to cling, naturally and simply falls away. Life is lived now, not by dictation, but in free, effortless unfolding. Our actions become truly constructive. Life unfolds freely ... it unfolds as The Tao.

Good Luck? Bad Luck?
Which is it … ?

An old man and his son worked a small farm, with only one horse to help with the plowing and the chores. One day, for no apparent reason, the horse bolted and ran away.

"Oh … what terrible luck!" the neighbors said.

"Good luck? Bad luck? Who knows which it is?" the old man replied.

Three days later, the old horse returned … with five wild stallions in tow.

"Oh! What **great** luck!" the neighbors exclaimed.

"Good luck? Bad luck? What's the difference?" the old man wondered aloud.

The next day, the son set about the task of taming the wild stallions. One of the horses threw him, and he broke his leg. He was now unable to help his father run the farm.

"Oh … what awful luck!" the neighbors said.

"Who knows if it's good luck or bad luck?" the old man asked.

Two days later, the army came through the countryside, looking for strong, young men to fight in a far-off war. They saw that the young man with a broken leg was of no use to them, so they left him behind and went on their way.

"What wonderful luck!" … the neighbors laughed and cheered.

The old man shrugged and went on with his work . . . .

Shortly after the army had come through the land looking for strong, young soldiers, they lost the war. The farm, and all it produced, was now the spoils of the victors. There was no one in the land left to ponder: "good luck? … bad luck? … which is it?"

Fear on the Meditation Trail
and
Remembering Virginia Myers

Perhaps the greatest gift we can offer to another being is freedom from fear. We can offer this gift only when we have first transcended our own fear. And we transcend our own fear, quite simply, by practicing the methods that make freedom possible. As we *live* this freedom, others see that freedom is possible. And, *if they are asking*, we can then offer to them the techniques we have discovered for realizing this freedom.

Yet, all too often, what is offered, when one is truly asking, is merely hollow assurance ... what I call "the bluff". This occurs when, for lack of knowing differently, we comfort others with empty words that only express the *hope* that our fears are unfounded. We pat them on the back and say things like, "There ... there ... everything is going to be fine. Don't worry. Everything happens for a reason. It's all going to be all right." The words may be true, but they're not spoken from the place of *knowing*. Reassurance comes only from the throat, not from the heart. The sentiments are void of wisdom.

However, it is possible to offer truth, assurance, and light from the place of *knowing*. True knowledge is realized, and fears are quelled, by *practicing* the ages-old techniques and methods that enable us to see through and beyond the illusions that are at the root of all fears. In time, and *with practice*, we begin to not simply *know*; we begin to even **know** that we know. It is probably the most comforting and reassuring experience imaginable! And when we *know*, no concept or idea ever again originates merely from a place of faith or belief ... rather, everything arises from the core of our very being ... from the place of wisdom. Truth has now become *who we are*. Truth, understanding and knowing radiate from us ... in our deeds and in our actions ... whether words are spoken or not. It becomes obvious. It is *felt* by those in our presence. However, simultaneous to arriving at the place of knowing, essential work must be done on the ego-self. For there is no place for arrogant or haughty wisdom. There can be no proselytizing. Confidence is assured when it is lived in quiet dignity. It cannot be forced. It's the greatest assurance possible to be in the presence of one who *knows* they know, because then we realize that the same freedom is possible for us, too.

It would be absurd to ask someone if they *believe* in gravity ... because we all experience gravity continuously. We feel it and see its results. It doesn't require belief because it is *known*. Of course, gravity is a phenomenon of the material, physical, world. It takes no insight ... no inner work ... to know the truth of gravity. It just *is*. So we are faced with a question: Is it possible to truly and fully and without doubt *know* at a non-material, non-rational, non-thinking level? Is it possible to *know* at the Soul level? Not faith ... not belief ... but *know*ledge! Is it true, as we have been led to believe, that everything at the Soul level must merely be accepted on faith? Or, must *anything* at the Soul level be taken merely on faith? If not, how can Soul-truth be *known*?

The great yogi of the 1920s, Vivekananda, once said: "There isn't anything that can't be known. But there is much that can't be known by the thinking, rational mind." Bridging the gap. How do we bridge the gap between the brain world of ration and senses, and the just-as-real, but non-material, spiritual world of the ethereal? I believe that Virginia Myers built that bridge. This is, in part, her story.

The Yin:

On a mild Autumn day in 1987 I received an invitation in the mail from a woman named Virginia Myers. Virginia was inviting me to sit Sunday mornings with a small group of meditaters who had evolved into The Tulsa Sitting Group. "The Group sits on Sunday morning for 45 minutes in silent, unguided meditation," the invitation read. I was intrigued, but I had not attempted to sit still and silently for 45 minutes straight since the early days of first working with my practice and the yogas. I hadn't persevered with extended sitting from the beginning, and mostly I remembered only that it was *awful*. (It was some time before I would discover the value of "awful" ... and even more time before "awful" became "exquisite".) Besides, by 1987 I had been teaching yoga for several years and, ego still firmly in place, I felt I had a reputation to maintain. What if I *couldn't* sit quiet and still, and at least *appear* focused, for 45 minutes? I decided to play it safe ... I discarded the invitation.

But invitations continued to arrive periodically. I didn't know Virginia Myers or know how she knew of me and my address ... although getting on mailing lists is neither odd nor difficult. As time passed, and invitations to sit with The Sitting Group continued to arrive, I began to find myself longing for a structured Sunday morning routine of some kind ... something far removed from the traditional. I was beginning to think this Sitting Group might just fill a void and deepen my work. So, I went ... and I sat. I discovered I *could* still sit for 45 minutes straight - still and silent - and I began to feel myself, ever so lightly, ever so slightly, begin to rest comfortably once again in that "inner place" (for lack of better words to describe it). It was a place I had read of and heard of and, indeed, had even *taught* about ... but a place whose truth and reality I had not personally *experienced* in all my years of working with just a Hatha Yoga practice.

Whether it was intentional on her part or not, in 1987 Virginia Myers began revealing to me the meaning of the phrase: "infinite possibilities". Or, perhaps put more accurately, she offered the space in which I could *find* infinite possibilities within myself. In fact, it's safe to say that I was unprepared for the breadth and depth of teachings Virginia Myers was about to offer ... teachings she apparently hadn't consciously planned, but teachings she had obviously planned *for*. My whole understanding of "infinite" and of "possibilities" was about to change.

I knew little of Virginia Myers' personal history, and was only mildly curious of who she was in earlier days ... before I met her. I had heard somewhere that, in the 1940s and '50s, she was a music teacher at The University of Tulsa and was influential in Tulsa's "arts" community. I didn't investigate, and didn't know if any of that was true or not. Virginia attended my yoga classes for awhile. And I knew that Virginia Myers was a kindly, thoughtful, insightful woman. She was probably in her late seventies when I first met her, and she offered her home and meditation/yoga room (an apartment-extension connected to the garage) to whomever wanted to use it. That was all I *really* knew. And it was enough.

For a few years, every Sunday morning possible, I made the drive to Virginia's house near the Tulsa Fairgrounds, quietly entered the meditation room, balanced comfortably (or **un**comfortably, as the case sometimes was! I was also fast learning to be unattached to comfort!) on my cushion ... and I sat. Following the breath. Abdomen in; abdomen out. Mind wandering; bringing the mind back to the moment. Exquisite comfort; exqui-site *dis*comfort. Focused, distracted. Discovering the experience of the senses. *Watching* ... for nothing in particular. *Finding* ... plenty!

I learned about the *senses* during those Sunday morning sittings. In the Wintertime: hear-ing the welcomed sound of gas jets igniting in the heater, the fan engage, and feeling glo-rious heat swirling about, warming the body. In the Summertime, hearing the welcomed sound of the air-conditioner and feeling the sensation of cool air swirling about, filling the room ... surrounding the body. In the Spring and Fall there were incredible aromas and cool breezes wafting through the open door and windows. Spring and Fall sensations seemed to originate *outside* of our little meditation capsule; in the Winter and Summer, sense stimuli came from *within* the meditation room. My understanding and discovery of sadhana (the teachings and reminders which arise sometimes in the unlikeliest of places) deepened ... in spite of my *personal* feelings toward what I was experiencing. I felt I was beginning to explore paths that had been tread and explored by the ancients since the be-ginning of time ... indeed, since the beginning of *timelessness*! All of this, I was soon to discover, was foundation for more profound teachings to come.

The Yang:

One day Virginia had a minor accident in her car and sustained a few cuts and bruises ... none of the injuries seemed to be serious. But there was a problem: her minor wounds would not heal. Tests were initiated. One test led to another. Finally all test results were in, and the results revealed that Virginia had cancer. More than just *had* cancer ... she was cancer-*ridden*. Cancer had metastasized throughout her body. Unbeknown, in the months and years that Virginia was routinely, but consciously, going about her daily rou-tine, cancer was spreading. She received some treatments of chemotherapy and radiation, but to no avail. It was too far along ... too advanced. Virginia suddenly found herself living, no longer on a tree-lined street near the Tulsa Fairgrounds, but now in the stark, fluorescent, steel and glass environment of an urban medical center. I went to see her often, and it was during those visits, I realized later, that my meditations with Virginia Myers *really* began.

I had never before had an opportunity to personally witness the results of years of extensive and <u>intensive</u> meditation practice. I had heard of it ... I had read of it ... but until that time, I had not personally witnessed it. I never really even thought much in terms of the *results* of a practice. I knew that it was important not to focus on results ... to just let results *reveal* themselves. Now I had the opportunity to see and hear, and to be in the presence of results revealed. It was an experience that, I think, comes to few of us in a lifetime. I embraced the opportunity that was offered me, and I learned to value the teachings even more deeply in the context of the flow of time.

Sometimes, when I went to the medical center to visit Virginia, I thought at first that I had walked into the wrong room. Changes in her physical appearance were so pronounced and so rapid, it was almost beyond belief. Of course, the chemo and radiation treatments had long-since rendered Virginia bald. While sitting and being with her, one could almost visibly watch her weight drop.

In those moments of just being with her, I began to understand the ancient axiom: "our body is what we *have*, not who we *are*". And I began to realize that, with all of the technological advances of the twentieth century, the profound truths first realized eons ago remain unchanged and completely, totally relevant.

If Virginia was affiliated with a formal religion, I never knew it. She was an avid student of philosophies and religions, but "captive" of none of them. She respected and understood the validity of any path that does not inhibit awakening. A fellow meditator and friend of Virginia's had given her a knit cap shortly after she entered the hospital. One day, as I was speaking with her, she suddenly put her hand on her now-tiny bald head and, with mock shock, exclaimed, "My god! Where's my cap? I probably look like some silly Buddhist monk!" Then her eyes became bright and lucid, and she laughed. I handed her the cap, she smiled a crooked, conspiratorial smile, put the cap on, and said, "I don't really mind so much looking like a monk ... but my head gets cold!"

After awhile, Virginia's communication became noticeably muddled and confused. She had great difficulty expressing the simplest of concepts. One day she made a garbled and completely incomprehensible statement. After speaking, she looked over at me in mock wide-eyed surprise and exclaimed, "*That* didn't make any sense at all, did it?!?!" And again, she laughed out loud ... laughed with the delight of a child indulging in the kind of silliness granted to a child ... expected of a child.

Another time, Virginia looked down at her bed sheet, which had the name of the hospital written in a geometric pattern. As if pondering deep in thought she said, "Now yesterday, these sheets had the hospital name written all over them." She studied the sheets closely; pulled back the spread and looked the sheets up and down. "Hhhmmmmm ...", she said, as if in a Sherlock-Holmes-detective trance. She studied the sheets more closely. Up very close ... then moving back and examining the whole bed. Finally I said, "Well, Virginia, the sheets *do* have the name of the hospital written all over them." She looked over at me with another sly smile of revelation and exclaimed, "Not to *me* they don't! I can't read *anything* today! It all just looks like so much geometric pattern ... no words there that I can see!" And again - the warm, completely untroubled laughter ... as if the discovery of life from the perspective of *leaving* the world is every bit as wonderful and fascinating and *perfect* as the discoveries and insights and revelations from the perspective of *entering* the world. She clearly didn't seem to distinguish between "coming" or "going" ... it was all just *discovery* for her ... and it was all *equally* wonderful. Where the discoveries fell on a linear time line of life seemed of no consequence to Virginia Myers. And her message in those moments seemed to be that they *are* of no consequence!

As more time passed, Virginia's appearance increasingly assumed the look of a newborn baby bird, or of a tiny mouse. She was becoming frail and tiny. Yet, wit, wisdom, and humor still flowed through her non-stop. This was obviously no act! ... not bravado! There was no way she was faking such lightness and genuine happiness day after day ... consistently ... *all the time*. Never a down moment. Never any melancholy. Certainly no self pity or depression. I realized Virginia was just *being here* ... that, for her, nothing of any real significance was happening. But what *was* happening for Virginia was wondrous adventure ... discoveries ... and intrigue. How it was affecting her body seemed of no particular importance to her. Most of the time she was just busy visiting with loved ones ... just like always ... like any other day. Of course, circumstances required the setting to be different from what she was accustomed to, but if that mattered to her, there was never any indication. "So what?", she seemed to be saying, "No big deal. **Really!** ... no big deal! And I *mean* it!"

There were some Sundays when Virginia was at home but she was too weak to come out to the meditation room and be with us. I had a key, so I would come early and open, and leave late and close. It saddened me that on some Sundays there were those who would not go into the house to visit with Virginia ... apparently unable to bring themselves to be with this deteriorating, tiny, shriveled form ... previously known as "Virginia". I understood their fear, for I, too, have much work to do to transcend attachments to form. More importantly, I knew that Virginia understood ... *fully* understood ... why they didn't come in to see her after the sitting. For she had transcended those very fears not too long ago herself.

The Work, I discovered is both *in* time ... and it's *out* of time. Being with Virginia Myers those last few months of her life made me realize the importance of creating and maintaining a practice *before* the drama gets too heavy. It enabled me to see that The Work ... **works**! That it's not just philosophy from the pages of some dusty old book. It's *real*! It's the very real work of consciously *embracing* real-world situations and predicaments, *embracing* real-world stuff, and eventually *transcending* that real-world stuff. Virginia had learned to use a thorn to remove a thorn ... and then, without a backward glance, she threw them both away.

Without the slightest noticeable effort, Virginia Myers taught the most valuable lessons, and offered the greatest gift ... the **greatest** gift ... that one being can offer to another: the gift of freedom. She taught ... and she *demonstrated* ... that absolute, total, and complete freedom is possible. That fear is just another hype ... just another illusion. She offered it in, ultimately, the only way it really *can* be offered: by personally being free from fear. Anyone in her presence saw it ... felt it ... *knew* it. It was so obvious! It was so simple.

Seeing Darkness

We don't drive around
admiring Christmas lights
at noon.
We wait until dark.

We don't sit and watch
a fireworks show
at noon.
We wait until dark.

It is the **darkness**
that lets us see the light.

Without dark,
there is no contrast.
Without contrast,
there is no vision.

Without light,
there is no contrast.
Without contrast,
there is no vision.

Light and dark
are the yin and the yang.

Vision is the Tao.

THE WARLORD

The Tao Ling Monastery had been under siege for several days by the fierce warlord Feng Lai. The monastery's defenses were few, and during this time many of the monks and students, who considered the siege to be the death-blow of the monastery, had fled through secret passageways to the hills and woods far beyond. To safety. Some were caught and brutally slain by the warriors who were driven, not by purpose or honor, but by greed and malice.

The old Master of the temple, Wong Fei Ling, sat in his small, simple quarters and calmly awaited the final outcome. He occupied his time with the practice of devotions and occasionally indulged in the jnana yoga of mathematical puzzles. His only protection consisted of a large bolt that secured the chamber gate from the rest of the monastery, and he knew that, in time, the large wooden structure would fall also.

On the fourth day of the siege, it fell. The warlord Feng Lai went directly to the quarters of the monk Wong Fei Ling. The warlord stood menacingly at the entrance to the little room ... a sardonic, sly smile on his lips. The little aging monk stood, too, beside his simple table, and faced the warlord who approached him with hatred in his eyes and death in his hands.

"Don't you know who I am?" Feng Lai shouted down at the monk. "I am the one who can thrust my sword through your heart without blinking an eye!"

"And don't you know who I am?" the little monk almost whispered. "I am the one who can take your sword through my heart ... without blinking an eye."

Looking for Truth
In All the Wrong Places

I was looking down … at leaves I was raking … at a yard full of leaves that seemed never-ending. I had raked the whole yard two days earlier, and now, looking at it, it was as if I had never even touched it. Two days after raking, the whole yard seemed to be right back where it had been. Then I looked *up* … into the trees … and it was obvious that the trees had much fewer leaves then than they had two days earlier. "I **am** making progress!" I thought, "I just wasn't looking in the right place! I have to look *up*!"

I was looking up … at a sky dark and gray and foreboding. The wind had picked up and the dark clouds were rolling in bringing the promise, or perhaps the *threat*, of a terrific storm. Such weather has a reputation: it's called "dreary" and "nasty" and "threatening" and almost any synonym for "bad news"! Then I looked down … and what I saw was green grass and brilliant flowers … all of which had been made possible by the season's "nasty" weather. "Progress **is** being made!", I thought. "I just wasn't looking in the right place! I have to look *down*!"

I was looking within … I was sitting in mediation and my breath was still and I felt surrounded by the warm gentle glow of peace. "Nothing can disturb now!", I thought. "I am 'one' with it all. Total inner bliss!" Then I opened my eyes and saw the suffering of the world. Not just huge dramas, like wars and pestilence and starvation (but that, too!), but just the everyday suffering that surrounds us all much of the time. It felt as if my peaceful refuge were a cop-out … as if I were hiding from the work to be done to relieve suffering wherever I can, wherever I find it – the Bodhisatva Vow. "There *is* purpose!", I thought. "I just wasn't looking in the right place. I have to look *outward*!"

I was looking outward … at all of the chaos and noise and bright, glaring lights … at the pain and suffering of others … at my *own* pain and suffering. And it seemed absolutely totally and completely and overwhelmingly real … as if nothing else exists … as if it's just day after day of misery, followed by death. Then I closed my eyes and focused my awareness on breath … on the gentle rise and fall of my abdomen as breath flowed calmly and gently into and out of my body … noticing how the gentle flow **calmed,** first my body, and then my mind. I could still hear all of the noise and suffering, and I could see all of the bright lights, but it was as if I were a steady flame surrounded and protected by cinderblocks. The chaos could not touch me. "There are possibilities!", I thought. "I just wasn't looking in the right place. I have to look *inward*!"

A Seer knows where to look … and, perhaps more importantly: *how* to look. For one who knows where to look and how to look, it is *all* real … it is all relevant … and it is all relative. There is no escape … no *need* to escape. For a Seer, there is no confusion in the mind over contradictions. For a Seer, this flows into this flows into this. There is perfect, seamless continuity …

BEING

(Birth, Death ... Beginning, Ending)

As each beginning is an ending,
so, too, each ending is a beginning.

The door that is marked "EXIT" on one side
and "ENTRANCE" on the other side
is yet the same door.

The birth of the baby is the end of the fetus, as
The beginning of childhood marks the end of infancy, as
The birth of adolescence is the death of childhood, as
The coming of adulthood signals the parting of adolescence.
Truly, the death of the body inspires the Birth of Spirit's Freedom.

"Death" is the name we give to a transition that our mind cannot *sense* ...
and our brain cannot comprehend.

The essence of Being is beyond time and space.

Birth is beginning *and* ending ...
as surely as death is both ending and beginning.

Being cycles forever on ... and on ...

What can we say to one we have left behind in a dream?
What can we say to one who is lost in dreaming?

Our responsibility is simply to be ... to *be* - simply.
And to share that be-ing ... by simply *being* it.

All else is Higher Law.
　　We can only flow gently with it,
　　　　and marvel at its beauty and perfection ...

　　... including what *appears* to be birth

　　... including what *appears* to be death.

Doing the Work

In W. Somerset Maugham's classic tale, "The Razor's Edge", main character Larry Darrel spends time in a monastery in Tibet. There he finds the incredible peace and serenity that he, and most of us, have been searching for most of our life. But one day Larry is told by one of the monks that the time has come for him to leave the monastery. He is shocked, stunned, and depressed by the news, but the kindly old monk tells Larry that it is easy to get holy on the mountain top, but it means nothing unless one can go back into the fire ... into the city ... into the day-to-day mundane realities of life ... and practice the teachings. So Larry Darrel leaves the monastery in the mountains and returns to Chicago ... just in time for the Great Depression.

In a similar story we are told of a monk who spent many years in the mountain caves ... meditating and praying and becoming one with the universe. He decides the time has come to return to the village he left many years earlier and share what he has learned. He returns to find many changes in his village ... not the least of which are electricity and motorized vehicles and more noise and more lights and more smells than he had ever known before. The monk boards a bus to make his way to the place he remembered the village church to be ... in hopes of working with the priests toward the goal of enlightening the villagers. But as he rides on the bus, the noise is incredible, and exhaust fumes come in through the windows, and the ride is rough and the people on the bus are jostled about, bumping the monk this way and that. Slowly the monk becomes edgy ... then the edginess grows to anger, and it is all he can do to keep from yelling at the people or leaving the bus at the first opportunity. It is then that he realizes the work he has to do was not *just* in the caves of the mountain, but just as truly in the village ... in the bus ... with all its overwhelming sensory stimulation.

Stories such as these remind us of the context in which we should relate to our yoga practice ... our yoga class ... our yoga room, with all of its environment-creating embellishments. And that is: the *real* work of yoga always lies *in* the world ... in the predicaments of urban existence and human relationships and interactions. It's easy to "get holy on the mountaintop" ... to close our self off in our room, in our meditation, and in our practice ... it's easy to live the day just waiting for and anticipating the glorious routine that awaits us, once we get home ... away from the horrors of the work and the people and the traffic and the noise.

It is said that the fire tempers the blade and makes it strong and sharp and able to keep its edge. So it is, too, with the fire into which we are thrust day after day after day. If we use our yoga practice as an escape, then we are merely going through the motions ... simply working with the body ... and missing the *essence* of yoga. The discoveries we make in the practice of the yogas are meaningless unless they are shared with others.

And they can only be shared with others if we are willing to enter into all environments ... where true suffering lies. And they can only truly be shared with others when we learn to *live* the teachings ... not preach them. And we can only live them *in* the world ... not in the cave.

"Your daily life is your temple and your religion," Kahlil Gibran tells us in "The Prophet". And it is only when we have *reached* the mountain top, he says, that we truly *begin* the climb.

Yet, these stories are not to say that the time in the "cave" ... the time in our yoga class, and our home practice ... are not very important and not to be enjoyed. Because it is in these ideal environments that we can experience the purity of our discoveries ... without the distractions of the world. It is here we can realize the *potential*. But the potential remains only that unless and until we take it with us into the office, into the home, into the car, and indeed into whatever setting we find our self.

The World Trade Center
and the Purple Flowers of Yellowstone

One day in 1989 I was sitting in an airport waiting room reading a magazine article about Yellowstone National Park. I remember it was 1989 because it was the year after the devastating 1988 fire ... a fire that charred and destroyed over 30% of the vegetation and wildlife in that massive park. Four pages of photographs were particularly memorable. Each of the pictures was taken from the same spot ... featuring a north, south, east, and west view. All four pictures showed mostly just charred, black wood, sprinklings of gray ash, and a deep blue sky. Black and gray and blue ... lots of black ... was all that comprised each picture. And all that broke the lines of black against blue was the occasional jutting, spiked remains of tree trunks and fallen branches ... scattered about, looking like the remnants of a war zone. One view showed a valley, extending to the far-distant horizon miles away ... black and gray all the way to blue. Another view showed a huge Rocky Mountain foothill in the near distance. The foothill was solid black. And the larger hills and mountains behind that one ... all black ... against a blue, cloudless sky. Each photo was shot with an extreme wide-angle lens that gave the viewer the sensation of standing in the very spot the photograph was taken. At the bottom of each picture one could see the ground, right *here,* in the photograph ... or lift the gaze up and see all the way to the cloudless blue sky. They were four of the simplest, most uncomplicated, least interesting, and most depressing, photos I had ever seen. I have loved Yellowstone since I first saw it in 1958. Seeing these pictures made me feel shocked and empty and sad.

The viewer's eyes were drawn to the horizon in each photo ... which accentuated the massive breadth of it all. However, if the viewer looked closely at the entire picture ... looked down to the bottom of each photo ... to where both viewer and photographer stood, there was something visible that was both stunning and impressive ... something that gave hope. It was something that, in fact, *filled* each of the pictures ... the width and the breadth, all the way to the horizon, but was obscured by the charred wood, and was invisible except when looking directly down at the very standing spot. Scattered about, between the myriad black charcoal and gray ash that extended infinitely in all directions, were tiny purple flowers, just beginning to make their way to the surface of the burnt carnage ... to face the sun and the elements ... to start the life cycle anew. Their stems were no bigger than a mere thread and the flower was not much larger than a pinhead. But they were a start ... they were a beginning. And they could only be seen from just the right perspective ... from the perspective of right *here.* Yet visible or not, here they were. They were right ***here***! They were just as much the truth of those photos as the charred landscape, the destruction, and the black and gray and blue.

Each photograph, when viewed from one perspective, showed a possible glimpse of what the end of the world might look like. And each photo, viewed from another perspective, showed what the *beginning* of the world might look like. The beginning of Life! Each photograph blended yin and yang into perfect Tao, when seen clearly … as most images do … when we are able to break free from the emotional binding around our heart.

Six years later, in 1995, I had the opportunity to visit Yellowstone. I even had the opportunity to stand in the very spot where those photos were taken. Now I looked in all directions and saw a veritable *sea* of wildflowers! In every valley and on every hillside were thousands and thousands of Rocky Mountain wildflowers. And thousands of tiny, bright green 3-to-12" pine trees were everywhere. The splash of color was dizzying and dazzling! All of the burned black wood was still there … but what dominated the vision now were the flowers and tiny pine trees. And the irony was that it was the black, charred, desolation ash that had made it all possible!

On September 13, 2001 I thought of those two days in two different years, linked by a common experience: a day in 1989, sitting in a waiting room, and looking at those magazine photographs of charred trees and ash; and of a day in 1995, looking out at an incredible panorama of new life that had arisen from that destruction.

September 13, 2001 was a Thursday … two days after the incomprehensible horror of the destruction in New York City and Washington, D.C on the previous Tuesday: September 11th. Each Thursday evening, as I have since 1986, I facilitate a yoga class at Tulsa, Oklahoma's St. John's Episcopal Church. Yoga is, above all else, a Philosophy of Being … being in the moment, and *how* to be in the moment. In each class I try to impart a relevant perspective on the philosophy of yoga … one that gives meaning to events, no matter how terrible the events. I was struggling that day with what to say … and how to say it. I knew that two days later many people's minds were still going to be focused on the tragic events of 9/11, and struggling to build some kind of bridge between the beautiful and simple philosophy of the Yogas … and the horrible, mindless destruction and hatred that all of the world had witnessed at The World Trade Center. Is yoga philosophy just pie-in-the-sky fantasy? Did the sickening images on tv reveal *real* reality? What good is some nice, sweet, rosy philosophy … in the face of the worst terrorist act of all time? These seemed to be the true questions.

Then, as with the photographs of charred Yellowstone, I began to "look down" … to look **here** … to bring my field of inner vision from the horrible images of crumbling 110-story office towers to the events that had followed on the heels of that horror, and brought us all the way from September 11th to September 13th … a mere two days later … but light years further! I began to realize that that afternoon's news stories had been *filled* with accounts of people, not just here in the United States, but **the world over** reaching out helping hands and a comforting embrace. Love … **love** … was pouring in with the same ferocious force with which those massive towers had crumbled to the ground just two days before. The very acts that were intended to buckle the knees and break the will were, instead, opening hearts. And once open, the pure love that knows no bounds was pouring out ... filling New York City ... filling Washington D.C. ... filling the world! Pure love was taking root in the charred remains of The World Trade Center as surely as the little purple flowers had taken root in the charred remains of Yellowstone National Park. The little purple flowers soon became a vast array of flowers, and then came the pine tree seedlings. And Life began anew. That's what the charred remains of Yellowstone came to. And seeing the aftermath of 9/11, we were witness *once again* to what the flowering of ***love*** comes to.

Heaven & Hell

A samurai warrior once asked a monk to explain to him about heaven and hell.

The monk looked the warrior up and down. A wry, condescending smile crossed his face and he asking, mockingly, "*You*?!?" "*You* want to know about heaven and hell? And you call yourself a samurai warrior?" The monk's tone grew even nastier. "You're so filthy I wouldn't hire you to fight for me if you were the last warrior in existence! You're insulting! Your sword is probably dull, and you smell as bad as you look!"

The warrior couldn't believe his ears! He became furious! First, a look of total disbelief crossed his face, then dismay, and finally total rage filled his being from head to foot. He was red in the face. His breathing came fast and loud. He began to draw his sword. He was so infuriated now that he made whining, squealing noises. He held his drawn sword directly over the head of the little monk, prepared to strike the fatal blow.

The monk stood motionless, expressionless. Casually he gazed into the eyes of the enraged warrior. He smiled gently now, and quietly he said, "That, my friend, is hell."

At first, the warrior scarcely heard the words through his fury, and they registered slowly. His shaking began to cease. The red drained from his face. His breathing calmed. Finally, he lowered and re-sheathed his sword. The warrior began to understand and appreciate the wise words and the bravery of the little monk ... that he would offer a teaching that endangered his own life. A broad smile spread across the warrior's face.

"And that," said the monk, "is Heaven."

****

Traditional assumptions lead us to believe that we must first die in order to experience heaven or hell. However, yoga wisdom tells us that heaven and hell are inherent in the moment ... and that the choice is *ours* as to which it will be.

NAMASTÉ

There is within each of us a place in which infinite wisdom resides. Regardless of how thoroughly that place has become cloaked and disguised by ignorance, confusion, fear, and anger ... its light shines eternal.

Given our circumstances, our knowledge, and our understanding, we are each doing the best we can to find that place and to offer it as a safe haven to others ... appearances sometimes to the contrary.

When we consciously reside in that place and look out at the universe from its perspective, and when we look in one another's eyes and see that there is only **one** of us, in individual manifestations ... we acknowledge that truth when we say:

*   *   *   *   *   *   *   *   *   *   *

NAMASTÉ

*   *   *   *   *   *   *   *   *   *   *

With eyes closed, visualize your arms extended before you. Imagine each hand holding a candle. Visualize candles of different sizes, shapes, and colors in each hand. And "see" that the candle in your left hand is lit; the candle in your right hand is not.

Now visualize bringing the wicks of the candles together so that the two candles share one flame.

Visualize holding the candles apart again. Are there now two *separate* flames? Or is there *one* flame ... in two *individual* places? For one who is aware, both answers are "*Yes*". Both truths exist simultaneously.

There is the *appearance* of separateness ... with the candle flames ... with us. But in fact we are each *individual* beings, not separate beings. We are the same essence of being, each with our own unique personal packaging. We occupy separate spaces and places. The word expressing the harmony of these confusing, yet not contradictory, realities is:

NAMASTÉ

The Breath
as Tao

As our practice deepens and we become increasingly quiet in the moment, we begin to discover that we are surrounded by teachings ... by sadhana ... and that those teachings are sometimes very subtle and very simple.

Consider, for instance, the process of breathing. It would be absurd to ask if someone prefers inhalation to exhalation. Obviously, we are equally dependent upon *both* for breathing to occur. Although the in-breath and the out-breath are opposites ... clearly, they are not in opposition. They are opposites in *harmony*! When we are conscious in the moment, the simple, essential, process of breathing "teaches" us the philosophy of The Tao: that, for anything – *anything* – to exist in the world, it is dependent upon its opposite for its very existence. *Everything* that exists in the world is dependent upon its opposite for its existence! There can be no up without down, no hot without cold, no left without right, no right without wrong ... no inhalation without exhalation. The simple process of breathing, when we are conscious of it, teaches us the profound truth of being ... the profound truth of opposites in harmony, that is expressed in The Tao.

For instance, the concept of "darkness" has a bad reputation ... "dark night of the soul", for instance. However, without dark, there can be no contrast. And without contrast, there is no sight. Likewise, without light, there is no contrast. Without contrast, there is no sight. If there were only light, there would be no vision. If there were only dark, there would be no vision. Both light and dark must blend in *harmony* for there to be vision.

Much, if not most, of our suffering occurs when we engage in the human tendency to cling to this and push against that. We often think to our self, "If only I could get more of this and have less of that, **then** I could be happy!" But it isn't having "this", or not having "that" that causes our suffering; it's the struggle we create – *we* create! – as we cling to "this" and push against "that".

The struggle ceases, and so does much of the suffering, as we begin to learn to move toward the positive without pushing against the negative. For instance, we learn to fully accept that there is, and there is always going to be, suffering in the world, even while simultaneously we begin the work of relieving suffering wherever we find it ... knowing full well that suffering is not going to go away. It's the paradox (but not the contradiction) of yoga: that we work to relieve hunger, for instance, knowing there will always be hunger. We work to end ignorance, knowing there will always be ignorance.

It's possible to discover these profound truths, not just by reading the great holy texts or being in the presence of great teachers ... but also by simply sitting with the breath, observing the breath, and being forever open to what the breath *reveals* ... beyond simply oxygenating the body.

Nothing Goes Away

There are many who come to a yoga practice thinking if they can just get more of this and get rid of that, *then* everything will be okay. They think they're going to learn how to eliminate something(s) and how to acquire more of something(s) ... all of which will *finally* lead to happiness. But yoga philosophy holds that we have *already acquired* ... that we are whole and complete just as we are ... and that the only thing we have to *get* from our practice is an understanding of how to use and understand what we already have ... what we already are. We begin to focus, not on *changing* the daily events of our life, but on *understanding* them.

Juan Matus, in the Carlos Casteneda books, advises Carlos that "nothing needs changing in a Luminous Being". As our practice deepens and we begin to increasingly discover who in truth we are ... our spiritual essence ... our soul-self ... it *seems* as if we are changing. But, in fact, we are simply *dis*covering what was already there ... what was always here. "Change" is the illusion; **discovery** is the reality. If we dissect the word "discovery" we find "dis", meaning to undo, and "covery", meaning to shroud or conceal. So when we dis-cover something we are merely ***un***-covering ... revealing what was always here ... what already exists. Nothing new is created ... except perhaps awareness.

An analogy I often use in class is: The Bright Light. As we sit with eyes closed, we visualize that before us appears a bright light ... a light bulb, fully exposed and shining brightly. Then we imagine as if shrouds or veils are being draped over the bulb ... each one increasingly inhibiting the light. These veils are labeled: ignorance ... confusion ... fear ... anger ... all of the negatives that tend to block our awareness of who in truth we are. Finally the veils are so many and so thick that the light is blocked completely, and we look around and wonder, "What happened to the light?" Yet it is not gone. In fact, it still shines as brightly as ever! But its radiance is blocked by the veils that we ... *we* ... have placed over the light, continuously, throughout the years. In our yoga practices, what we are doing is systematically removing ... peeling back ... the shrouds that block our light. Gently, slowly, one at a time, the light begins to reveal itself. The light that was *always here* begins to shine brighter and brighter ... illuminating not only *our* way, but helping others to find their way, also.

Our practice is not about *getting* something ... or getting *rid* of something ...it is about discovery. It is about revealing. It is about finding what was always here.

Non-sense ... No-body ... No-thing

Most of us have spent a lifetime in what noted American yogi Ram Dass calls "Somebody Training". We are proud to be a "somebody" ... and no one wants to be a "nobody"! But then, our relationship to these concepts begins to change.

As our practice deepens and our awareness heightens, we begin to discover that the work we are doing in yoga is not of the senses. It *involves* the senses, but it is not literally "sensual". We begin to realize that the world of the senses is limited to the physical, mundane world ... it is the world we experience during most of our daily, waking consciousness. However, in our practice of Raja Yoga and the various meditation techniques, we learn to quiet our attachments to the senses and realize that the information the senses provide, although very helpful, is also very limited. It is from that vantage point that we begin to discover that the practice of the yogas is literally "not of the senses" ... that it is **non**-sense. Our practice is literally nonsense! ... constructive, meaningful, nonsense.

Also, as our practice deepens and our awareness heightens, we begin to discover that the body is what we *have,* not who we *are*. We discover that we are *not* a body ... we are soul-essence, atman, spirit-self ... that just happens to be inhabiting a body. We are not a body. We are "in the body, but not *of* the body", so to speak. Thus, from the yogic vantage point, we are literally **not** a body. We are no-body. We are *nobody*! And yet, we *are*!

Likewise, we live in a world of things. Our body is certainly of the world of things. However, we also discover, as our perspective changes, that who we truly are is not of the world of things. We are **not** a "thing". Thus, we are also no-thing. We are *nothing*! And yet, we *are*!

It might seem strange to think that our practice is "nonsense" and that one of the goals of our practice is to discover that we are "nobodies" and "nothings". And yet, these yogic discoveries ... these realizations ... truly mark milestones in our practice, in our understanding, in our transition of illusions, and in our realization of wisdom.

Hierarchy

There is a tendency, with those doing the work on themselves, to see goals and accomplishments in terms of hierarchy … "higher" self and "lower" self … all of which simply leads to more value judgment. The assumption is that the world in which we live, including the body with its mind and senses, is of a "lower" world … that it is somehow inferior, and that if we can just persevere, with hard work and luck, we can transcend this repulsive world and catapult the self into a higher realm … into the higher self.

When conducting classes I seek to avoid terminology that reinforces such polarizing concepts. Rather than referring to "higher" self and "lower" self, I use phrases such as "the obvious self" or the "worldly self" … the self of matter and of the senses … and the "subtle self" or "soul self" … the self of spiritual/soul essence. Our body, mind, and senses, for most of us, makes up the world of the "obvious"; while our Spirit Self and innate Wisdom constitute the world of the subtle. Many of us are not aware that we already *are* spiritual essence and that we already *have* wisdom … that we already *are* wise. It's an important distinction! It's the distinction between having to get something vs simply *discovering* what one already has. It's the difference between being, and knowing, we are whole and complete, or thinking we're lacking.

In addition to teaching yoga classes for many years, I have also taught a form of *jnana* yoga, called "math", at Tulsa Community College and elsewhere. A student, not accustomed to getting right answers, suddenly solved a rather complex problem one day and exclaimed, "I'm becoming a genius!" I suggested that perhaps he was simply discovering the genius that was always his. A genius that had been blocked by his *belief* that he didn't have it to begin with. He was not *getting* … he was *dis-covering*.

It isn't that the goal is to leave "lower" self behind … while taking refuge in "higher" self. "Yoga" means "union" … joining together … harmonizing … opposites existing, not in opposition, but in complement … and as one begins to "yoke", one experiences that the worldly self of matter and possessions and change and time and space indeed *complements*, does not oppose, the self of soul essence, and wisdom. Nothing is gained (except *awareness*) and nothing is left behind.

Breathing Into
The Head ... the Heart ... the Throat

Two crucial practices of yoga include: breathing exercises and visualizations.

The breathing exercises accomplish more than simply oxygenating the body. When coupled with visualization practices, one is capable of directing, managing, and controlling the energies of the body, and thought energies of the mind. Also, visualizations enable one to gently, but firmly, hold the mind in the moment. We all have a mind that tends to wander ... to drift into nostalgia and future projections and get preoccupied with things that others said to us and the general human melodramas that make up daily living. So when we practice breathing exercises, or stretching and twisting exercises of the yogas, we also practice focusing *awareness* on both the sense-sations that we are experiencing, and also on those places in the material body, and the ethereal body, that we wish to influence.

The heart is the symbol of compassion in the body. It is not where compassion *"is"*, but rather, where it is physically symbolized. In order to deepen a sense of compassion, when we practice the breathing exercises of yoga, we may choose to visualize the breath being drawn directly into the heart ... as if the chest has nostrils ... as if we are literally breathing into the heart and exhaling from the heart. For instance, to reinforce our sense of inner strength, we may visualize that on the in-breath we are drawing directly into our heart center ... heart chakra ... all of the pain and suffering and fear and anger and bigotry of the world, and that we are exhaling in its place the love and compassion and understanding that is ours to offer. Knowing now that we have nothing to fear from the world's negatives, we may consciously choose to work directly *with* those things ... as we seek to convert negative energy to positive ... to compassion ... rather than continuing to *avoid* those things.

The head is the symbol of reason, logic, and intelligence in the body. It is not where intelligence *"is"*, but rather, where it is symbolized ... just like compassion in the heart. In order to deepen a sense of reason, when we practice the breathing exercises of yoga, we may choose to visualize as if the breath is being drawn directly into the crown of the head ... as if there are nostrils at the crown of the head, and that we are literally breathing *into* the crown of the head and exhaling *from* the crown of the head. To reinforce our sense of ration and logic, we may visualize that on the in-breath we are drawing directly into our center of reason all of the ignorance, confusion, fear, and anger of the world, and exhaling in its place the understanding and comprehension that is ours to offer. Knowing that we have nothing to fear from the world's ignorance, we consciously choose to work directly *with* those things ... as we convert negative energy into understanding.

Like a social worker who makes a conscious choice to work in the poorest, most dangerous, part of town because they know that they have the innate positive energy necessary to offset the negative energy in their midst. They make a conscious and deliberate choice to walk straight into the lion's den. As one's sense of compassion and understanding strengthens, one becomes truly fearless. Not in the sense of reckless bravado, but *truly* fearless ... knowing that there is truly nothing to fear! Knowing that, although the body may be vulnerable, the self is not!

However, there is a danger in resting too fully in the heart. It's possible to become mired in compassion. If we rest too fully in the heart of compassion, we become like someone encountering another who is stuck in quicksand: in a zeal to help, they simply jump in. Then there are *two* who are caught in suffering ... neither is capable of doing anything about it. And there is a danger in resting too fully in the head. It's possible to become mired in intellect. If we rest too fully in the head of reason, we become like a bureaucrat. Others come to us in genuine need, and we simply hand them a form to fill out ... never looking up ... never seeing who we're serving.

Therefore, in yoga we seek always *balance*! We seek to create balance between the heart of compassion and the head of reason ... that we may learn to be reasonably compassionate and compassionately reasonable. We create this balance by visualizing breathing directly into and out of the throat. As if there exist nostrils in the throat, and we are literally breathing *into* the throat and exhaling *from* the throat. The throat center ... chakra ... is the approximate physical mid-point ... point of balance ... between the head and the heart. We breathe into the throat and visualize breath energy flowing from the throat into the heart ... and, on the exhalation, flowing from the heart and out of the throat. On the next breath, as we breathe into the throat, we visualize breath energy flowing from the throat into the head ... and, on the exhalation, from the head and out of the throat. We may visualize this breath energy flowing *simultaneously* from the throat into the heart and head, and *simultaneously* back out again. These are techniques designed to bring our heart of compassion into balance with our head of reason.

We often hear it said, "Listen to your heart" ... "follow your heart". However, we have a head for a *reason*. It is not enough simply to be caring; nor is not enough to simply be knowing. One must seek always to be *In Balance*.

Planting a Seed

Westerners often conceptualize "accomplishment" in a linear way. That is, when something is *done,* it is *accomplished.* And, indeed, with most things worldly, that is how it works. That's how bridges are built and degrees are earned and one achieves success. Therefore, it is sometimes difficult for a student of the yogas to grasp the concept that in order to "accomplish" in the work of maintaining a practice, one must learn the art of doing - ***nothing***! ... but, doing nothing *consciously*! Because, in the practice of the yogas, it is not our objective to make something from nothing, but rather to discover what already is! It's like planting a seed ...

We can't grow a plant! It's not within our power to grow a plant. We can't reach into an acorn and extract a trunk and branches and leaves and assemble them and make a hundred-foot-tall tree from an acorn. But what we can do (and *all* we can do!) is create an environment in which the tree *can* grow. We can plant the seed, and we can water the soil, and we can fertilize the soil ... providing nutrition. We can create and enhance the environment in which the tree can grow ... but we can't do the actual *growing* of the tree.

Thus it is, when we practice the yogas ... when we establish the setting, with candles and gentle music ... when we stretch and twist and practice the breathing techniques of the pranayams ... when we work with meditation ... what we are doing is simply creating the environment in which we can discover what is *already accomplished.* We are not becoming wise; we are discovering our wisdom!

I advise students not to look for results, because if we look for results, the results are rarely soon enough nor quantitative enough, nor are they always what we expected they would be. Rather, I tell them, seek simply to create an environment in which the results can *reveal themselves*! With the practice of the yogas, there truly are results; however, it is important to understand that they will reveal themselves in time and with patience. Sometimes the results turn out to be just what we expected them to be. Sometimes the results are *nothing* like we expected. Sometimes they are *just* what we expect ... and more. Sometimes, if we lack knowledge of our wisdom, it may even seem as if the results are a disappointment ... and students without sincere motivation may get discouraged and abandon their practice.

It is important to simply establish a practice and work with it ... and work with it ... and work with it ... just because it's what we do! By so doing, we plant the seed. Then one day, perhaps much to our surprise, we see a frail, vulnerable seedling just breaking the surface. And while the seedling is young and vulnerable, we may seek to protect it from the forces that would destroy it ... reinforcing our practice by surrounding ourselves with encouraging books and beings. In time, and with commitment and intent and practice, one day we discover that our practice is a Mighty Oak ... straight and strong and tall and no longer in need of a protective environment or special care. It is capable of withstanding fierce winds and prolonged draughts. And it began with the mere planting of the seed!

The First Time …
Again!

An old proverb in Tibet says that we can't walk into the same river twice. Even though the river retains the same name, and may *look* the same year after year, the fact is, like everything else in existence, it is in a constant state of flow and change. It does not *stay* the same … not even for a minute. Even a stagnant pool of water is constantly changing. Therefore, it is said, we cannot walk into the same river twice.

And by the same token, we can't truly walk down the same street twice. We can't even talk to the same person twice. In fact, we can't even breathe into the same body twice! Consistency is the illusion … change and flow are the reality. So each and every time we do something, we're actually doing it for the *first time … **again***!

Doing something for the first time *again* may sound a bit like the idea of regaining our virginity, or turning back the clock. However, if everything in the world is in constant change and flow, then in truth, we never actually do anything twice. Each and every thing we do, each and every time we breathe, each and every time we sit or stand or speak with someone or wash a dish or mow the lawn or meditate … we are truly - and **literally** - doing it for the first time … *again*!

Understanding this gives one a whole new perspective on such concepts as "repetition" and "boredom". After all, boredom is simply the ego self's demand that the moment have something more … or at least different … than it has. The ego self is never satisfied with the moment as it is, because it always thinks that the moment should be somehow different than it is. But as the True Self begins to see through the illusions that the ego self is incapable of comprehending, then experiences such as boredom become absolutely impossible! If each act is, indeed, new and unique … and being done for the very first time *again*! … then, from that perspective, boredom is not even possible! As we begin to rest more and more in The True Self, and less and less in the ego self, each moment and each act, regardless of how similar it may be to previous acts and moments, is endlessly fascinating … endlessly interesting … is being done *for the first time **again***!

Shapes

Consider the shape of water.

Cup your hands and dip them into a pool. Lift your hands from the pool and look. Notice the shape of water.

Tilt your hands and let the water run over your fingers and into a vessel. Look and see the shape of flowing water.

Look at the shape of the water within the vessel. Let the vessel of water sit for a few days and see how the water disappears from its container. What is the shape of water now?

Look in the air and see the shape of water vapor … formless … invisible … yet, still ever present in the sky … water in the shape of clouds. Watch the clouds as they fall back to the earth as droplets … the shape of water is now rain. Or see the shape of water as it falls back to earth as snow … or ice.

See the shape of water as it flows in a stream. The water in a stream appears to be one thing … one thing called "stream" or "river" or "creek". Try to cut the stream with a knife. Throw a rock into the water and try to break its shape. Or burn the water with fire. Try to push it back upstream. Try to clutch a handful of water in your fist. Split the stream in two enabling each part to flow in a different direction … making two streams from one … creating two shapes from one.

Now consider the shape of Soul. Soul is like water.

Look in a mirror and see the shape of Soul … shaped like its vessel … its body vessel.

Like water in a glass, the Soul assumes the shape of its vessel. Form changes with changing circumstances, situations, conditions, and time. Yet Soul remains as is.

Like a stream, Soul flows. Like a pond, it rests. Like a mirror, it reflects. Like vapors rising to be clouds, it is invisible … and yet it is. Then, as mysteriously, it *becomes* visible once again … as clouds. It eludes touch and yet it is filled with substance.

Soul returns again to form. Like water falling back to the river. Back to the pond. Filling human form once again … and again. Filling human form so completely and so convincingly that it seems at times as if it really *is* the form itself.

Soul, like water, is shapeless. It *takes* shape. It *becomes* shape. Yet a mind that sees no deeper than shape and appearance easily confuses shape for substance.

Be as unconcerned with the form of Soul as you are with the shape of water. Each is formless … each is potentially *all* forms. Rest comfortably in the fabulous mystery of the shape of the formless.

Turbulent River

The mind is often like a raging, turbulent river. Sometimes a practice is terminated because one is unable to quiet the mind. However, if we think of the mind as being like a river ... sometimes raging, sometimes deep and calm ... we discover that we don't have to stop it. All we have to do is **watch it**!

We have the option of standing on the bank and simply watching it!

What we create with our practice is the ability, the power, to swim through the raging torrent to the bank. Once on the bank, we realize we can't stop the river, and we don't have to. We are free to simply sit and watch. Just *watch* the river ... simply marveling at its qualities. We can even *appreciate* its nature ... including its rage!

If we happen to see someone stuck in the river ... caught in the torrent ... helpless in the swirling current ... we are now able to offer them help ... *if* they want it. Whether or not they accept our help is *their* choice, but we are obliged to offer that help, and now we can, because we are safely out of the swirling turbulence. We are safely on the bank of the river. We can choose to go swimming whenever we want.

Returning from the Deaf:
Noise and Distraction

If yoga and meditation mean "being *in* the moment", then are distractions even possible? If whatever is "distracting" us is just what is in the moment, then how could we possibly be distracted *from* "what is" *by* "what is"? And yet, we are. Or, at least, we perceive that we are. A jet flies overhead; a motorcycle goes by; we hear people talking and laughing nearby; or perhaps the worst: someone's cell phone rings! Are we distracted?

It is incredibly easy, when working with our practice, to keep pushing for the ambiance … to become attached to the setting and to creating and maintaining the *perfect* setting … the candles … the incense … the music. And then something interferes with that … and we're caught again! We're had by *us*! We know setting and ambiance are not what it's all about, and yet there's no denying that a peaceful setting *helps*! It helps us to rest in that place of inner peace and to become rejuvenated and reenergized.

Here's an exercise in perspective that I sometimes suggest in class: Imagine that, for no known reason, you were to suddenly lose your hearing. It's just *gone* … and you're plunged into silence … total silence. For several months you live in silence, and then one day, also for no known, apparent reason, your hearing just as abruptly returns. It's back! You can hear everything again!!

Now, imagine how you would *relate* to that experience! Imagine how you would perceive each and every sound. You own voice; the sounds of crickets on a Summer night; water splashing; the voices of loved ones. Every sound, regardless, would be a symphony! It wouldn't matter if it were the sound of a cell phone ringing or a door slamming … every sound would be Heaven!

When we are ***truly*** at rest in the moment, we hear each sound for the first time … *again*.

This is it!
The Spiritual Experience

There are those who come to a yoga practice in search of a "spiritual experience". To those seekers I say: *This is it!* This *is* the experience of Spirit embodied!

The body is the instrument that enables Spiritual Self to express itself to other beings, and to relate to other beings. Otherwise, we are like a radio without a signal. The signal is real; the signal is absolutely essential ... and the same can be said for the radio. However, without the radio, the signal is worthless. And without the signal, the radio is just furniture. It cannot manifest communication. The relationship between signal and radio, Spirit and body, is truly symbiotic ... each is dependent upon the other for its meaningful existence.

To the one who is in search of the Spiritual Experience, I say: *This is it* ! Each and every thing we do, each and every expression of the Self ... whether good or bad, passive or active, peaceful or violent, caring or apathetic ... and each and every thing that happens to us ... whether we like it or not ... is truly a Spiritual Experience.

This
is
it!

Embracing vs Clinging

The open mind *embraces* concepts and ideas … and is always open to change … and is perfectly comfortable with the possibility of being totally and completely wrong! The embracing mind seeks only truth and is unattached to being "right".

The closed mind *clings* to beliefs and cannot fathom the possibility that the truth may in any way be different from its preconceived notions. The clinging mind holds fast to being right at all costs.

Gandhi once planned a huge march and demonstration. All plans were in place, when suddenly he realized that the dangers involved might vastly outweigh anything positive the march might accomplish. So he called it off. His colleagues and the organizers were confused and disheartened! They tried to "reason" with him, telling him that people had already made personal sacrifices to participate in this demonstration and he couldn't simply halt it at this late date. Gandhi replied, "My commitment is to truth … not to consistency."

Gandhi understood perfectly the distinction between embracing and clinging.

Yoga and Being

The being that is in time and space must come to harmony with the being that is timeless and spaceless. This is the work of the yogas. This is the work that we have to do.

Yoga means "union" … it means coming together … harmonizing. We know what it means to be *dis*membered; yoga means becoming *re*membered.

One of the most useful phrases in understanding yoga is: "**at a level**". In our existence, there isn't just one thing happening exclusively simply at the level of the senses. It isn't that simple. It isn't that *drab*! That's why, as our awareness deepens, we begin to experience metaphors all around us. We *swim* in metaphors!

When we're driving down the street, we're not *just* driving down the street. When we're interacting with another being, we're not *just* talking to them.

Every worldly act that we perform is a metaphor for something unfolding at another level of our being … simultaneously. And all that is occurring within inner levels of our being is being expressed at the worldly level through our actions, our thoughts, and our words.

The predicament for many of us is that we have consciously existed exclusively at the material level for so long that we have come to believe *it* to be absolutely real. Thus, we hear such phrases as, "I'll believe it when I *see* it" and "*seeing* is believing". We have come to live almost entirely in the senses and to relate only to the senses. Many of us have lost touch with what is literally the sense-*less* … with the self that is timeless and spaceless and yet is just as real as the mind and the body.

We are a "self" that is timeless and spaceless and *im*material. We are also a "self" that is embodied, material, and very much in time and in space. Both of these selves are real. And both of these selves must discover the way to exist in harmony. The methods of yoga enable one to find that way … and to find that harmony.

Self Esteem:
A Field of Flowers

One sunny Spring afternoon I was driving across a prairie in central Oklahoma. The prairie was like an ocean ... vast as the eye could see, in all directions, waves of gentle slopes and valleys ... simply fading into the horizon. And the entire prairie was covered with a small yellow flower called Black-eyed Susan ... a sort of miniature sun flower. There were thousands ... tens of thousands ... maybe *millions* ... of bright, yellow, identical Black Eyed Susans. I crested a small rise, and beyond I saw more ... and more ... and more ... ! It was incredible! Who knows how many acres ... square miles ... of seemingly **identical** wildflowers surrounded me, for I could only see to the horizon in any direction, and every time I peaked a crest, there were more! And then I realized ...

Of all of those thousands, maybe millions, of Black-eyed Susans that covered acre after acre after acre, not one of them ... *not one!* ... had refused to open and radiate its brilliance and aroma because it felt lost in the crowd. Not one of them had refused to open because it felt irrelevant, insignificant, or insecure. Each one of those millions of wild flowers was simply doing what it does: following its dharma ... doing what it does simply because *that's what it does*!

As we progress with our practice, and as we begin to discover who in truth we are and what it is we do (our dharma ... our path ... our purpose), then we become less preoccupied with recognition and accomplishment and achievement, and more focused on simply doing what it is we do ... as well as we can possibly do it.

Our ego-self, still intact but less relevant, now takes a backseat as our yoga-self discovers our purpose and allows the doing to simply flow through. We become more like the wildflower of the field, and whether we're a "cog in the machine", or a "number", or a one-of-a-kind eccentric artist, becomes less and less important. Like a finely crafted violin, we become less preoccupied with *creating* music, and more focused on simply letting the music flow through.

Perspective

Our initial motivation for creating a practice may be *change*. We may think that something about us or our surroundings is inadequate … lacking … in need of our improvement. We may become preoccupied with what yogis call the "if onlys": if only I were taller … if only I were shorter … if only I were younger … if only I were older … if only I had more money … if only I lived here … if only I lived there … on and on and on. We almost all have our list of "if onlys". And when we focus on our "if onlys" our practice becomes focused *out there* … we become preoccupied with trying to change objects and things and other people and settings and circumstances. We soon discover we are climbing up a sand mountain … the harder we struggle, the harder the climb, and the more we just slide back down. Nothing gets accomplished.

However, as our practice deepens, we begin to discover that it isn't our circumstances that have mired us down in emotional quicksand; rather, it's how we *perceive* our circumstances … our environment … our "givens" … how we relate to them … or don't. As our practice deepens, the focus of our work begins to shift from "out there" to "in here". We begin to realize that our goal is not *accomplishment*, but rather discovering that which *is* accomplished! What already is … who we already are! We discover that the goal of yoga is not so much doing as it is *discovering*! The work of yoga is *discovering* … *un*-covering … revealing what already is. Not creating something from nothing, but discovering creation!

One fine day we discover that all that changes is our *perspective*. And all that changes is … *everything*!

To someone looking back at us, as we move through the course of our day, it may seem as if nothing much has changed. But from where *we* now rest … consciously "in here", looking "out there" … nothing is the same!

Picking Apples

One of many sayings in The Book of Tao (pronounced: "dow") advises us to see things just as they are, without *wanting* them to be otherwise. At first glance, this appears to be a statement of apathy … of blind acceptance. But it isn't. The operative word is "want" … "without **wanting** things to be otherwise". This doesn't mean that we observe a situation, shrug our shoulders, say "ho hum" and walk away from it. It doesn't mean that we don't do anything about it. It means we accept it just as it is, and then do what is within our power to *positively* affect it.

Take, for example, a visit to the doctor. If the tests the doctor runs reveal a serious condition, the doctor and the patient don't enter into a conspiracy to pretend that nothing was discovered and everything's fine. Rather, both doctor and patient *accept* the situation as it is, without wasting valuable time lamenting the fact that things aren't different. They set about doing what they can to positively affect the condition, the situation, and improve it or eliminate it … if possible.

If, when walking down the street, we see someone genuinely suffering, we accept the situation just as it is … and then **do** what we can to help alleviate the suffering. We don't simply shrug our shoulders, say "oh well … fate", and walk on. At least, if we're a conscious being, we don't do that. If we are being yogic, we fully accept their suffering, and then *do what we can to relieve it.*

Imagine standing on a ladder … under a tree … picking apples. Our basket is hooked to the side of the ladder, we pick an apple, inspect it, decide whether or not it is edible, and then either place the apple in the basket or discard it. We don't *judge* the apple. We don't judge the worms that are in it, nor the bruises rotting it. Rather, we simply decide if it is useful for our purposes or not, and based on that determination we place the apple either here or we put it there. Based on discriminative thinking, we do this or we do that.

There are no "bad apples". After all, what sane worm would bore into a "bad" apple? We accept the apple just as it is, and then act accordingly.

In the Moment

In the province of Wi Lu there lived an artist … an old woman by the name of Ling. Every morning Ling would search the streets and alleys of her small village for bits of broken glass, pottery, and attractive pebbles that she would collect in a bag and take back to her house early in the afternoon. She would use these small bits of rubble to continue her work. The townspeople wondered, to themselves and to one another, "What is that old woman up to now? Why could she possibly want those broken bits and pieces? Surely she is crazy!" But they called her "crazy" with an accepting smile, for the townspeople loved this eccentric old woman, and they protected her and bought her works of art, whether or not they understood them. This enabled her to continue to live in the village with them.

Near the province of Wi Lu there was also a temple of monks. One day the Master of the temple said to the student, Kwai Khan, "I want you to go to the artist Ling. Do not disturb her, stay at a distance, and simply watch as she goes through her morning ritual in the village … and then, again staying at a distance, follow her home and observe as she works on her art." Kwai Khan asked, "May I know why I am to do this, Master?" And the senior monk said, "If you observe closely, you will learn from the actions of Ling the secret of happiness." So early the next day, the young student journeyed into the town. He soon found the artist Ling at the edge of a village street, looking closely for bits and pieces to place in her bag. Young Khan observed from a distance and followed the old woman around the village as she searched and gathered, searched and gathered.

In time, Ling began to realize she was being observed. She approached the boy and asked, "Are you following me around town young monk?" "Yes, I am," answered Kwai Khan. "Have you nothing better to do with your time than to follow an old woman around the village as she scavenges for trash?", she asked with a smile. The boy replied, "My master in the temple said that I should watch you and observe … that by doing so I would discover the secret of happiness." At that, the old woman threw back her head and laughed so hard she almost dropped her bag of shards and pebbles. "Surely your master is playing a joke on you, young monk! But if this is the way you wish to spend your precious time, then by all means, please observe …" And the artist Ling resumed her search as if the boy were not present. Kwai Khan watched.

Early in the afternoon, just as always, the artist Ling ceased looking and began the short trek back to her meager dwelling … a one-room hut that rested on sand at the edge of the desert. Once there, she walked to the rear of the hut where there was a table, upon which were the tools of a sculptor, and next to the table stood a mound of clay, as tall as the old woman herself. The mound glistened in the sun as if it were a huge diamond! The sparkles were an array of all of the colors of the spectrum. The boy knew not what it was, but he was impressed with its strange beauty. Ling poured the bag of broken bits out on the table, went to the mound of clay, and with a bucket of soft, moist clay, she began expanding the large, glistening shape. Then, while the new clay was still moist, she painstakingly pressed into it the shards of broken glass and pottery and the tiny pebbles. When she was done, she stepped back and looked with approval at her accomplishment … for the expanded mound now glistened even more brilliantly in the afternoon sun. She smiled her satisfaction at Kwai Khan, who smiled back his appreciation of this … this … well, he didn't know what it was, but it was truly beautiful! And he loved to simply stand and stare at it; it seemed to come alive in the changing sun.

Ling walked over to Kwai Khan and stood next to him. "Do you see in my creation the secret of happiness?", asked the old artist. "No," said the young monk, "I do not. But it is beautiful!" "I tell you," said the artist Ling, "your master at the temple is playing a joke on you. I know nothing of the secret of happiness. I go into the village each day and I collect what I find on the ground and in the gutters. I collect those things that others see as rubble … and I bring them back here and arrange them in my … in my …", the old woman looked down at the boy and laughed, "I don't know what it is, either!!" And they laughed together … but neither could deny the beauty of the decorated mound. Then she looked compassionately down at the boy and said, "I know nothing of the secret of happiness, young monk. I know only how to do each day's work … one moment, one movement, one breath at a time. I focus not on the outcome of my work, for I am an artist. I don't know when it is done until it is done. I let others decide what it means. I simply *do* … I create … one moment at a time … with no concern for the end result. I simply do each task as it arises … one moment, one movement, one breath at a time."

Freedom

Two things
every mind must discover:

It can want
and not get,

It can not want to do
but still do.

This is called Self Control …
It's called Self Discipline …
It's called *Freedom*!

There are many who think they cannot do something until they *want* to do it and that, conversely, if they want to do something, then they *must* do it. Many believe that what meditation and yoga should teach them is how to eliminate their wants and desires. But, in fact, what meditation and yoga teach us is to *honor* the mind and all of its predicaments … including its wants, desires, dislikes, fears. … while at the same time discovering that those things are simply the predicaments of the mind. They do not have to be *our* predicaments. They don't have to go away, nor do we have to follow their dictates. All we have to do is become aware of them, observe them, discover their nature, and discover the power that they *don't* have over us.

I can want a candy bar … and simply choose to not get one. I can want a drink … and simply choose to not pour one. I can not want to mow the lawn … and mow it anyway. I can not want to go to work … and go anyway.

Yoga and meditation mean:
Doing our duty …
Being responsible.
Being *free*!

Light On the Path

A map shows the way;
a light reveals the way;
the path *is* the way.

Yoga is a light on the path.

Without a consciousness-enhancing practice, it is as if we are standing on the path ... but it is midnight ... no moon ... no stars. We are left with no choice but to grope our way down the path in the dark, making slow progress, wandering off the path frequently, and struggling to find our way back.

As our practice deepens, the moon becomes full and bright. We can at least get an idea of where we're going and how to get there ... but obstacles, as well as realities, are still obscured and distorted because the light is low. But we practice ... and we practice ... and the full moon of night becomes the dawn of a new day, and as our way, and everything surrounding our way, becomes increasingly clear, we look around in wonder and amazement at all that is revealing itself to us.

What we're seeing is what was always here. But now there is light on the path!

Black Elk

Black Elk had a vision on a mountain top. After he returned to the village and told the people of his vision, they were filled with questions ... not so much about the vision itself, but about the particulars preceding it ... seeking to discover what *led* to the vision. They wanted to know which mountain he had stood on, which direction he faced, what he was wearing, what time of day it was ... for they, too, wished to have a vision. And they believed if they could recreate all of the particulars perfectly, then perhaps they too could be so blessed.

Black Elk patiently answered all of their questions. After he had done so, he told them this: "However, none of that matters. What mountain it was ... where and how I stood ... the time of day ... none of that matters. Because, you see, *every* place is the center of the universe."

Discovering Wisdom

Wisdom isn't an accomplishment.

Wisdom is what we discover. **Dis**-cover … **un**-cover..

All we're doing in our practice is *dis*covering what is already there.

What is already here.

Who we already are.

We Carry it With Us

Shortly after arriving home from a visit to Hawaii a friend asked me, "Couldn't you just *feel* the spirituality of Kauai?" I had to agree that, indeed, I could!

"But," I told her, "that's because I took it there with me. I felt it just as surely in the plane on the way over … and in the airport before boarding the plane … and in the car on the way to the airport."

A given place may complement our spiritual center in such a way that we confuse *what* we're experiencing with *where* we're experiencing it. But it isn't the place. It's us. We carry it with us. We always have.

The Music and the Jackhammer

Our predicament is akin to this:

It is as if we decided to play our favorite music on our stereo. And as the music is about to play, just outside our window a construction crew begins using a jackhammer. The construction noises are so great we can no longer hear the music ... even though it continues to play. In time, we adjust to the noises of the machinery, scarcely noticing them anymore ... the music we had decided to play is now long forgotten. Then something happens. The workers take a break. The noise stops. And there is the music ... the music we had forgotten all about ... it had been playing all along, but we couldn't hear it, and we hadn't heard it for so long we had completely forgotten about it!

This is roughly the predicament we face with hearing our higher mind ... listening to our inner voice. Our senses have become like a jackhammer ... keeping us so distracted at a worldly level that we can no longer hear the "music" of the Soul ... the music that is always there, always with us.

With our practice, we learn to release attachments to the senses ... to still the mind ... that we may hear what Quakers call "the small, still voice within". It's always there. It's always here ... constantly advising, re-minding, and guiding. All we have to do is create the *environment* that it may be known ... known and discovered. As a band aid, we can turn off the jackhammer for awhile, or build a sound-proof booth against it ... but once the wisdom of the inner self is *known*, and the inner silence is felt, it no longer matters whether it's the jackhammer or the music!

A Glimpse of Kundalini:
The Fourth Chakra Opens

Visualize a vast, grassy field. It's Wintertime; the grass is yellow-brown, and everything *looks* lifeless ... although we know it isn't. Visualize the same field now in early Spring. The first flowers of the season appear ... jonquils and crocuses. The days may still be cold and gray, but color begins to appear in the field. Soon, tulips bloom, the jonquils and crocuses settle back into the earth, and the grass turns a luscious green. Flowers of Summer - black-eyed susans and crepe myrtle - replace the flowers of Spring. And although the first of the flowers to appear are seen no more, we know they aren't "dead" ... for reappear they will - the next season - and the next - and the next.

Like eyes blinking ... the lids close, yet vision isn't lost. So it is with the Awakening of Kundalini. The word "Kundalini" literally translates from Sanskrit as "coiled". The image is of a coiled serpent, resting at the base of the spine (Sushumna Nadi), awaiting its journey through the Chakras ("centers") of awareness. But the serpent is simply a symbolic image to assist one in visualizing and understanding the awakening process, the process of becoming aware: aware of being ... aware of meaning ... aware of LIFE.

Kundalini Yoga (also known as Laya Yoga) is the yoga affecting the Divine Power (Kundalini Shakti), the seven centers of spiritual energy (chakras), and is the yoga responsible for arousing the dormant Kundalini symbolic "serpent" as it rises to unite with Lord Shiva (total consciousness) in the Sharasrara Chakra, located at the crown of the head. All seven centers are pierced by the passing Kundalini Shakti (energy) as it rises up Sushumna Nadi on its journey of awakening. As each chakra is aroused, awareness expands, and the practitioner begins to live life **simultaneously** at all levels of being. All is transcended ... yet nothing is left behind.

As the Serpent Power rises in Sushumna, awareness envelopes all of existence. What we once thought to be the whole of reality becomes just pieces in a vast mosaic ... vision moves back and back and back, like the effect one observes with the increasing range of a wide-angle lens ... we begin to see more and more ... and the Picture of Purpose expands to include this ... and this ... and this ...

Prior to the awakening process, it's as if we're playing a game of Cosmic Hide and Seek. First we "hide". We enter into the world and immediately family and friends and teachers help us create our worldly universe ... albeit, inadvertently ... based almost entirely on the senses and mundane "knowing". We enter into, and in most cases embrace, a reality that says "seeing is believing" ... the senses are real. We pass through what famous American yogi Ram Dass calls "somebody training". We become *somebody* ... collecting identities ... layer upon layer upon layer. One of the first, and most powerful, of the identities is our name. We hear it in a crowd, it gets our attention ... because "Richard" is *who I am*! Someone says my name and I respond, "Hello! Are you addressing *me*?" That's *me* all right! And we collect other identities along the way ... some of them transient and changing from moment to moment, some of them with us for life: son, brother, student, profession, intelligent, good-looking, fat, thin, American, humanitarian, caring, insensitive, warm and compassionate, or cold and unfeeling ... on and on and on ... all of them earthly, worldly identities. All of them ultimately transient, of course, so if we get too attached to these identities, we suffer. Time passes and things change, and we watch the identities fall away and collapse around us. We see it often: someone retires from a profession and no longer knows who he or she is: "If I'm no longer a _____, then who *am* I?!?!?!?!"

The chakras (a Sanskrit word meaning, literally: "wheel" or "center") symbolize the various levels of consciousness and awareness one experiences on the journey through life; although they may not all be experienced in one lifetime. There are seven chakras in the Kundalini system of yoga, ranging from the most primal ... mere physical survival – chakra one ... to full awareness of the Spiritual Self – chakra seven. All of these levels of being already *exist*, but as our practice deepens, we become increasingly aware of them.

Other chakras/energies focus on sexual prowess and power acquisition ... situated in the body in the region of the sex organs and the abdomen (the sun center ... the *solar* plexus), respectively. The first three chakras, for the most part, manifest in most people already "active" ... manifesting as the will to survive, to reproduce, and to control one's environment - including the people in it. But sometimes, along with age and growth, comes some degree of insight. *In* – sight. A phenomenon of yoga occurs that is sometimes referred to as the "opening of the fourth chakra". First we've hidden ... now we begin to seek.

The fourth chakra is symbolically located in the human heart ... manifesting as compassion. One begins to realize there *is* more to life than just getting and controlling what we want ... that there are *others* in the world, indeed, who are more *like* us than unlike us, and we have responsibilities to them. As the fourth chakra opens, we begin to see and experience the interrelated qualities of all things ... to see The Big Picture. We have the fascinating experience of vision expanding outward, while simultaneously turning inward. On the journey of awareness, I personally find Fourth Chakra Awakening to be one of the most exciting experiences imaginable! It's akin to the experience of driving across endless prairie to the Rocky Mountains, and then suddenly rounding a bend and seeing them before you for the very first time! There they are ... in all their majesty and grandeur! Or traveling to the ocean, topping a rise, and suddenly looking out on a vast expanse that's almost too much for the mind to grasp. It's the experience of re-birth ... what some might call being "born again". It's discovering and *knowing* that we are not alone! It's the discovery that not only is there "something more", but also the realization that we haven't even started yet ... that the discoveries are just beginning!

In the 1980s I worked for a computer manufacturer in Tulsa, Oklahoma, and had an experience many of us have had: I found myself working for someone who was mean, vindictive, conniving ... who would do whatever it took to try and undermine my self esteem and create a setting in which I would, hopefully, want to resign. One day, I sat at home, brooding over the situation, realizing there was *nothing* I could do to win this person over, and pondering: "Why me? I don't deserve this! I don't want to fight with anyone. I just want to get along and do my job. Why have I been singled out for this kind of treatment? I do as good a job in the department as anyone! Why me?" Then the fourth chakra opened and I could see it all from a different perspective ... from a whole new angle. I remembered that my boss had once told me of relationships in the past ... two former spouses and a father who had been physically and/or psychologically abusive, and of a current spouse who was milquetoast and listless. I remembered that the three abusive influences had all displayed characteristics including being intelligent, driven, assertive, independent, and self-motivated ... all traits that also seemed *to* characterize *me*! But there were significant differences: although I was assertive, I was not aggressive. Although I was energetic and enthusiastic, I was not "driven". I was independent, but not to the point of being uncaring. On the surface, I appeared to have all of the character traits of others who had threatened my boss. So the natural reaction was to lash out quickly and furiously, and do what was necessary to eliminate this perceived threat ... i.e., *me*. When the situation was seen from the *personal* perspective, why I was being treated this way seemed to make no logical sense. But when viewed from the Fourth Chakra ... big picture, *im*personal perspective, it made **perfect** sense! I was ultimately fired and escorted from the building by two security guards. It was an unpleasant experience, but one I at least understood perfectly.

T. S. Eliot described this awakening of Fourth Chakra Awareness when he wrote: "At the end of my journey, I find that I am back where I started. But it all looks different." Sometimes I conclude a class with: "All that changes is our perspective. All that changes is *everything*."

As our fourth chakra opens, we also become aware that most people are still functioning primarily at the level of the first three chakras: survival, sexuality, and power. Therefore, it is essential that we take with us, on our journey of awareness, a healthy dose of wisdom ... lest we become mired in judgments of others. Our awareness ... our understanding ... of the Cosmic View deepens with experiences like these. Cosmic Hide & Seek. Seeing the Spark ... catching a glimpse of the Light. Seeking becomes *discovery*!

"I am never disappointed by the actions of others because I expect nothing from them."

Sri Yuketeshwar

117

WORK

"It's a five-o'clock world," The Vogues' sang in their 1963 hit. "It's a five-o'clock world when the whistle blows, and no one owns a piece of my time."

The extent to which we segment our life … categorize, label, and isolate … goes far beyond just our personal identities of who we think we are. What we experience, how we experience it, and all we perceive in the moment we call "the day", is subject to, and determined by, the mind's never-ending pigeon-holing … evaluating, judging, comparing, and creating. Of all these experiences and categories, probably none is more heavily laden with negativity and judgment than the one we call "*work*".

"Up every morning just to keep my job," sing The Vogues, "Gotta find my way through the hustling mob."

Say "How are you today?" to someone on a Monday morning and notice the response you get. Ask the same question on Friday and notice the difference! On a Friday, eyes beam wide, a broad smile splits the face, and the response is often an exuberant, "It's Friday!" … as if that says it all … as if to say, "Once again we have survived the preceding horrid four days. We suffered through the week and *made it to the weekend*!"

We know the distinctions. We know them by heart. For it is, after all, the heart of confusion that created the distinctions in the first place … and their coincidental suffering. We know when we're "at work", as opposed to being "at home". There's no confusing being "at work" with being "on vacation". We know which is "our time", and who "owns a piece of our time". Leisure time? Work time? We know which is which … clinging to one and resisting the other. And we both envy and scowl in disdain at those who seem to actually *like* their work. We sneeringly call them "workaholics".

And yet, maybe there is another way to perceive the distinctions. There are those who have discovered that when we're "at work" there is perhaps no better opportunity to be of service … to offer our being to other beings. Author Jo Coudert, in her wonderful book ***Seven Cats and the Art of Living****,* observes that, "Work is what humankind has supposedly been cursed with since the days of Cain and Abel. It is what people plan to escape from into retirement. It is why people play the lottery or scheme to make millions in the market … so they will no longer have to work. The ideal setup has become to have to do as little work as possible. But," Coudert continues, "I have found that work is the meat of life. It is the part you can sink your teeth into, and from which you get real nourishment." Is it possible that we have slipped this far from perceiving work as service … as yoga … as Karma Yoga … as a genuine avenue to true bliss?

"The word Karma," Juan Mascaro writes in his introduction to the Bhagavad Gita, "is connected with the Sanskrit root Kri, which we find evolved into the English word 'create'. Karma is work, and work is life." And in the text of the Gita, Krishna tells Arjuna: "Set thy heart upon thy work, Arjuna, but never on its reward. Work not for a reward,

118

but never cease to do thy work." Krishna is not telling Arjuna that work should be without reward, nor is he telling him not to accept a reward for work; rather, he is telling Arjuna to not let reward be the *purpose* of work. Further, he inspires Mascaro's words when he tells Arjuna that "to avoid work is to avoid life".

How exhausting it is to be forever in the presence of the negative work attitude that is so pervasive in our contemporary culture! In addition to facilitating yoga classes at Tulsa Community College, and elsewhere, I also teach basic math at TCC. I find the work, the environment, my colleagues, and the students to be, almost always, delightful and a pleasure! Yet I find the same T.G.I.F. consciousness there as truly as any other place I have ever worked. That attitude has simply become a thoughtless habit for many ... but what a debilitating habit! And I find I must frequently ask myself, "What is *my* role in all of this? What are *my* responsibilities?" I can't get angry with them for doing this to themselves; that would just fan the flames. I can't reveal the ignorance of their ways, as most of what I would say would be meaningless in the context of their world, and would only anger and alienate them.

The Vogues sing: "Sounds of the city pounding in my brain, while another day goes down the drain." Sounds pretty hopeless! Yet from another perspective author Anne Morrow Lindbergh writes, "What a release it is to work in such a way that one forgets oneself, forgets one's companion, even forgets where one is or what one is planning to do next ... to be drenched in work as one is drenched in sleep or drenched in the sea."

Which will it be? It can be either, of course, depending on who we are and how we choose to perceive our world, and how we choose to perceive our roles and responsibilities, and how we choose to perceive the *expression* of those roles and responsibilities. We **choose** how we perceive our world! It is so easy to forget that we have *choice* ... so easy to sink in the quicksand of traditional perception ... so easy to come to believe that Fridays are superior to other days, in much the same way as we have come to believe that rainy days are "nasty" days, but warm, sunny days are the "beautiful" ones. Indeed, it's almost as if we've forgotten we *have* choice and rein over our happiness!

"Work," wrote the poet Kahlil Gibran, "is love made visible."

The purpose of work, in the context of yoga, is *service*. "Service," St. Thomas Aquinas observed, "is the highest form of prayer." Jesus told his disciples that as they did, in service, for others, they did also for him. Thus, the Wise Ones tell us: work is service, and service is the highest form of prayer; work is love made visible, and God is love.

If the Grace of Work isn't obvious from a personal perspective, perhaps it's time we try working with another perspective. For whether our work is merely what we must endure to make it to retirement or to the weekend, or whether it is the setting in which we share our being with other beings, not by preaching or arguing or trying to convince, but just by *being* ... this is **our** choice! Drudgery or service, heaven or hell ... the choice is ours. The choice is *always* ours! For how we perceive work is, after all, a function of how we perceive one another ... and how we perceive our *self*.

We Exist …

first,
to find the true self …
the Spirit self …
the Soul essence …
the being that is nameless and,
thus, has many names.

We Exist …

second,
to share that being with others
simply by *being* it.
Not by preaching.
Not by debating.
But simply by *being* …
by being *simply*.

All else …
the stuff of the world …
the stuff of life …
the melodramas of the day …
all become method …
technique …
means toward that end.

Nothing … Everything

As we sit
with eyes closed,
we gaze passively into the void.

We look for nothing;
we find everything.

Our vision, with the intensity of the sun,
pierces the fog of illusion.

We see clearly and truly,
perhaps for the first time.

We see all the way …
to *here*.

Just Notice ... Just This

In the practice of Vipasana, we passively observe the moment and what the moment holds ... without judgment ... without expectation. We practice letting the constantly judging, evaluating mind rest ... that we may, for a change, see things truly, see things clearly ... see the moment just as it is. We ...

Just Notice

What we begin to discover, as we rest passively in the moment, is that the truth we are seeking is with us always. It's with us always because it is inherent in us ... it's part of our packaging ... it isn't an acquisition, it's a discovery. All we have to do to find it is practice calming the mind ... quieting our attachments to the senses. The present is enough. The moment is everything. The truth of the moment is ...

Just This